A BELLEVUE LITERARY PRESS PATHOGRAPHY

PALE FACES

The Masks of Anemia

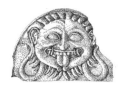

D0171056

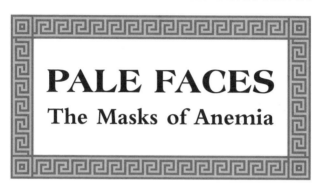

PALE FACES
The Masks of Anemia

CHARLES L. BARDES

Drawings by Barbara Kilpatrick

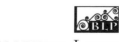

BELLEVUE LITERARY PRESS
NEW YORK

THE BLP PATHOGRAPHIES SERIES

With *Pale Faces: The Masks of Anemia* by Charles L. Bardes, Bellevue Literary Press launches its *Pathographies* series, each volume of which will chart the impact of disease on human individuals and populations from the biological, historical, and cultural perspective.

This series is dedicated to the memory of Lewis Thomas, author of several critically acclaimed books of popular science including *The Lives of a Cell: Notes of a Biology Watcher* and *The Fragile Species*. His longtime association with the New York University School of Medicine, beginning in the 1950s, influenced and inspired generations of young physicians, some of whom went on to become writers.

First published in the United States in 2008 by
Bellevue Literary Press, New York

FOR INFORMATION ADDRESS:
Bellevue Literary Press
NYU School of Medicine
550 First Avenue
OBV 640
New York, NY 10016

This book was published with the generous support of Bellevue Literary Press's founding donor the Arnold Simon Family Trust, and the Bernard & Irene Schwartz Foundation.

Library of Congress Cataloging-in-Publication Data

Bardes, Charles L., 1956–
Pale faces : the masks of anemia / Charles Bardes. —1st ed.
    p. ; cm.
Includes bibliographical references.
1. Anemia. 2. Anemia—History. 3. Anemia—Cross-cultural studies. I. Title.
[DNLM: 1. Anemia—history. 2. Anemia—psychology. 3. Health Knowledge, Attitudes, Practice. 4. History of Medicine. 5. Medicine in Literature.
6. Mythology. WH 11.1 B245p 2008]
RC641.B37 2008   616.1'52—dc22   2008006366

Book design and type formatting by Bernard Schleifer
Manufactured in the United States of America
ISBN 978-1-934137-10-9
1 3 5 7 9 8 6 4 2

I have cut up mine
Anatomy, dissected
my self, and they
are gone to read upon
me.

distortions on Donne, Meditation IX
"Medicamina Scribunt"

This is *Natures nest of Boxes*; The Heavens containe the *Earth*, the *Earth, Cities, Cities, Man*. And all these are *Concentrique*; the common *center* to them all, is *decay, ruine*; only that is *Eccentrique*, which was never made; only that place, or garment rather, which we can *imagine*, but not *demonstrate*, That light, which is the very emanation of the light of *God*, in which the *Saints* shall dwell, with which the *Saints* shall be appareld, only that bends not to this *Center*, to *Ruine*; that which was not made of *Nothing*, is not threatned with this annihilation.

—JOHN DONNE, *Devotions Upon Emergent Occasions*,
Meditation X, "Lentè et Serpenti satagunt occurrere Morbo"

pilgrim at plow

—Piers Plowman

Contents

Propylaeum

MODERN MEDICINE PRESENTS ITSELF AS A FORWARD MARCH of rational, scientific, progressive enlightenment, a triumph of fact. But beneath this bright and cheery tale lie darker layers of myth, alchemy, magic, ritual, oracle, memory, forgetting, fear, and melancholy.

Anemia is not exactly a disease but rather a core medical idea, like fever, that spans the world's many ages and its many places. How a culture comprehends this deficiency of blood, among the commonest of all human afflictions, bespeaks its concerns, its science, and its mythos.

The complete biography of a disease would unfold both its rationalized knowing (science) and its other-mediated knowing, which takes the form of folkloric, literary, religious, symbolic, and vatic expression. Also its poems, whether lyric, epic, ode, or dithyramb; also its unknowing.

Preface: Anemia

ANEMIA, ANEMIC, NO BLOOD, BLOODLESS, A DEFICIENCY OF blood. My life's blood is deficient.

Anemia is a doctor's number, rendered by a machine. Anemia is a man's pallor, his weakness, his fatigue, his sickness. I feel weak, I feel myself less a man, my manhood slips away, my lifeblood slips away, so this is how it is, living less, someday living not. The number half-records the sensation and half-predicts it, a foretaste of future dying, also a forecast. The physician speaks and listens, the blood count speaks, too, to him.

Anemia is a new idea, born of the instruments and later the machines that measure the properties of a person's blood. Anemia is an old idea, touching all we think and feel of blood, all we have ever thought or felt, here or elsewhere, now or before. Anemia aligns pairs of opposites: strength and weakness, vigor and lassitude, ruddy and pale, hearty and sickly, lively and moribund, robust and sallow, active and passive, virile and effete, sanguine and melancholic. Blood is life, lost blood is lost life, spilt life, anemia.

Blood circulates within the vessels and the heart, within the flesh and the organs, constant motion, life. Blood sits tranquilly under the microscope.

This book is an excursion, riff, or romp through the many cultural, literary, mythological, ritualistic, historical, and to some degree biological aspects of the medical condition *anemia*. To avoid cluttering the pages with footnotes, the references occur in endnotes that are an integral part of the text itself. These mean to add to the reader's pleasure, not to spin about academics. I invite readers who like this sort of thing to look at them from time to time.

Is anemia the sickly feeling a patient experiences, or the cells seen by a microscopist, or the number a machine prints out, the doctor interpreting the number, the patient hearing his number related, the construction of anemia, its history, its story, its understory, its fictive representations, its memory, its linkages, its metaphors, its allegories, its ceremonies, its concrete indication of disease or death? Its *alieniloquium*, its other-speak? Would a complete account not include all these things? If you prick us, do we not bleed?

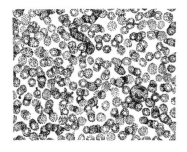

I. SYMPTOMS / I FEEL SICK

A symptom consists in feeling unwell. It is a subjective experience in which the body reports to the mind, or the mind to itself, that something seems amiss. Pain, fatigue, sadness, and a thousand other ills, all are symptoms that a man first registers within himself, then describes to a physician. Between the physical instigation of the noxious stimulus and its representation in the mind lie filters that are modulated by a person's private experiences, cultural contexts, and the dialogue with the physician.

1. Diseasification

A SEVENTY-FOUR-YEAR-OLD MAN VISITS HIS PHYSICIAN. HE feels well. His physical examination is normal. The physician orders blood tests. One of them is abnormal. The hemoglobin level is slightly below the normal range. He has anemia.

There ensues a great series of medical tests. He undergoes additional and numerous blood evaluations, then colonoscopy, upper endoscopy, upper GI series, and bone marrow biopsy. The doctor refers him to a gastroenterologist and a hematologist-oncologist. Each performs more tests, which are all normal.

What does the anemia *mean*? Mild anemia is not *itself* a problem, since no one feels unwell from mild anemia. The physician instead is concerned that the anemia may signify the presence of a disease that causes anemia. Some of these diseases are serious, and the tests the physician orders are intended to find if such a thing is present. The tests look for colon cancer, stomach cancer, prostate cancer, leukemia, and a great deal more.

And what does the anemia mean to the patient? Well, to find out, you'll have to ask him. And then you learn that he was fourteen years old when his father died, of an unidentified lung ailment, probably cancer. The men in his family die young, and he has always had a premonition that he too would die young. The youngest of three sons, he had a middle brother who died of pancreatic cancer in his forties, and an older brother—the man closest to him in all the world—

who died of leukemia in his early seventies. A favorite sister-in-law had recently died of lung cancer. These three deaths were all physically painful, debilitating, and degrading.

To the patient, the anemia means that his long-held premonition was coming true, and that he has a fatal illness, probably leukemia or cancer. As it turns out, the tests show that he is perfectly well. But the physician harbors a lingering doubt that some serious condition must be present. The patient senses this doubt and harbors it too.

He changes his plans. He decides to retire from his part-time job as a teacher, which he has hitherto enjoyed. He contemplates moving from his quirky old farmhouse into a retirement community, with nursing home options. He consults his lawyer regarding insurance plans that will protect his savings against estate taxes when he dies.

A healthy, vigorous, and rather upbeat man has been brought down a notch. His whole vision of life, and his expectations for the future, have been laid low.

What is this anemia? How is it defined? What does it mean? To *whom* does it mean? Is the meaning different among different participants in the drama: above all the patient and the doctor; and then the widening circles that surround them, the family, the clinic, the hospital, the insurer? How does the meaning change during different historical periods, and at different places?

Asking differently: What is anemia? What is anemia to us? Who is us? Which us? Now or when, here or where, present or other?

ANEMIA: WHAT THE DOCTOR IS THINKING
For the physician, anemia relates somehow to a lack of blood. The patient has had a test. The result is abnormal. He has anemia. Either he is not producing enough red

blood cells, or he is losing them too rapidly. We must perform further tests to determine the cause. I must notify the patient and order the tests. I must ask him some extra questions. Is he bleeding? Have his stools changed? Has he lost weight? I must explain, more or less. He will worry. Time is short. Others are waiting. What is wrong? Did I do something wrong? Did I overlook anything? Was he pale? Is he going to be okay? Someday not. Am I going to be okay? Someday not.

ANEMIA: WHAT THE PATIENT IS THINKING

The doctor called. I have anemia. Something is the matter.

What do I know about anemia? It has to do with iron, yes, or B12 shots. I should eat spinach (a fiction of early newspaper comics, based on a scientific paper's misplaced decimal point, then repeated in film and later in television cartoons. Spinach doesn't provide much usable iron, Popeye the Sailor notwithstanding.). I should eat liver (a fiction of early biomedicine, when liver extracts were used to successfully treat the hitherto fatal pernicious anemia). Or could I be sick? Anemia makes you pale, sick people get pale, the dying Ali MacGraw became pale from leukemia in *Love Story*, Mimi became pale and cold from tuberculosis in *La Bohème*, *"Che gelida manina."* Uncle Earl needed transfusions when he had cancer, and then he died.

The doctor said I could be bleeding. Maybe I have a bleeding ulcer. He asked if I was losing weight. What was he getting at? Maybe I have cancer.

A week passes.

I had the tests, they were all normal. I still have anemia, but it's not my iron or my B12. Now there must really be something wrong. The doctor said I need more tests.

More tests, procedures, X-rays, consultations, a week, two

weeks, a month. Colonoscopy—the specialist passed a tube through my anus to examine my large intestine—normal. Upper endoscopy—a tube down my throat to examine my stomach—normal. Chest X-ray, normal (well, some old smoking-related changes—are they okay? what exactly did he mean?). Upper GI series—I had to swallow a chalky liquid, it disgusted me somehow, though it tasted all right—results normal. CT scan—again the chalky liquid, again the nausea, again normal. Capsule enteroscopy—I swallowed a camera—normal. Visit to the hematologist-oncologist. Why does the doctor want me to see an oncologist? He must think I have cancer, he's not telling me. More blood tests, a week passes, normal. He wants to do a bone marrow biopsy. He has me lie down on a table and he puts a big needle in my pelvic bone to remove a sample of bone marrow; he sends this to the laboratory. He schedules a visit for next week—the follow-up visit for test results, must be serious. We sit in his office, and I have brought my wife. The test was normal. He wants to monitor me. I should come back in three months.

My brother George had anemia when he was younger than I am now, and then he needed transfusions, and then he got leukemia, and they gave him chemotherapy, and he got better for a while, and then he died. My brother John had cancer at forty, the doctors said they could do nothing, they monitored him, he died. My father died when I was fourteen, he sickened and died, they said it was his lungs, they never knew why, he was gassed in the Great War, a casualty of war postponed by twenty years. I think he must have had cancer, but they never found it or they never told him or they never told us, they didn't look hard enough but now they are looking at me, in me, through me.

Now I am sick. I must be sick, I have anemia, I don't feel bad, well I guess I am a little tired, well what can you expect. Again I am lonely, again unknowing and alone.

2. Pallor

ANEMIA IS BOTH AN OLD AND A NEW IDEA. ANEMIA IS BLOOD-lessness, a deficiency of blood.

Blood deficiency could be observed in two ways. First: you might see a person bleed. Hemorrhage is dangerous, hemorrhage may be fatal, to lose blood is to die. Blood is life, bloodlessness is death.

Second: a person might appear pale. The normal red color has left the cheeks. This pallor may be persistent or transient. Persistent pallor means a sickly life, on the one hand, or an indoor life, on the other. Sickly pallor is *wan, pasty, ashen*; indoor pallor is *fair*. The starvelings, waifs, and consumptives of the nineteenth century, and of its novels, are wan. So too are the oversensitive and overdelicate. But the young ladies in *A Midsummer Night's Dream* dispute which of them is fairest, for a light complexion then signified a life of ease and leisure. (The opposite obtains now, when *otium* wears the dark complexion of suntan, a fashion whose introduction in the 1920s is generally attributed to Coco Chanel.)

The pale maid is chaste; taken to the extreme, perhaps barren.

The scholar is pale: an indoor imputation, tinged with effeminacy. Bartleby is pale, and so is the critic William Hazlitt, "a pale anatomy of a man, worn and wan with study," and so are Kafka's anemic bank clerks. So too is the amorous beau, as in Suckling's seventeenth-century song:

Why so pale and wan, fond lover?
    Prithee, why so pale?
Will, when looking well can't move her
    Looking ill prevail?

The expression "pale and wan" as a trope describing the lover, especially the newly and suddenly smitten young man, has a long history in English literature, stretching at least to Chaucer, in the fourteenth century, and Robert Greene in the sixteenth.

Nor does Galen, the great physician authority of the second century, think highly of such men. "Their whole bodies were soft, white, hairless, fatty, lacking in veins, muscles, and blood."

And for Hamlet, all too famously, "the native hue of resolution / Is sicklied o'er with the pale cast of thought." More than three hundred years later, the American architect Louis Sullivan, champion of the skyscraper, castigates "the pallid academic mind."

Transient pallor: the cheeks blanch suddenly. Fear, pain, shock, apprehension, hearing bad news. Paris suddenly encounters Menelaus on the battlefield before Troy, the prince is frightened, and

As one who sees a serpent in a gully
starts back and steps rearwards, his limbs
trembling, his cheeks seized with pallor,
so did Paris fall back among the massed lordly Trojans
in terror of the godlike son of Atreus.

The Hippocratic texts of the fifth and fourth centuries BCE echo the simile: "the sudden sight of a snake causes pallor." Or: Odysseus strings his great bow, and the false suitors change color. In *The Odyssey*, Fear itself is pale.

Moses Maimonides, the great philosopher, scholar, physician, and leader of the twelfth-century Jewish community in Egypt, makes the same clinical observation. "When a man with a powerful frame, a sonorous voice, and a radiant complexion hears sudden news that greatly afflicts him, one can see his face turning pale, the glow dimming, the body hunching, the voice faltering, and when he tries with all his might to raise his voice, he is unable to do so, his strength is weakened."

Fear and eros may verge perilously close to each other. Dante's Paulo and Francesca, drawing closer and closer to adultery as they read of Lancelot and Guinevere, lament that "many times that reading impelled our eyes together and caused our faces to pale."

A frightened man turns pale, but encouragement may restore his color. Thus Shakespeare's Henry V enheartens his troops on the eve of Agincourt:

That every wretch, pining and pale before,
Beholding him, plucks comfort from his looks.

The physiology of pallor: either blood flow to the cheeks has diminished, or the blood that does flow there has too few red blood cells. The latter is what we usually mean by anemia. The former is a matter of circulation and is served by that elusive word "shock." Hemodynamic shock means that the blood pressure is dangerously low. The body shunts blood away from the skin and limbs to preserve circulation to the vital organs. Emotional shock causes a sudden stimulus to the sympathetic nervous system, the "fight-or-flight" response, and the body again shunts blood to the vital organs. In both situations, the cheeks turn pale.

Bleeding too causes pallor. The Hippocratic text *Epidemics* asserts that "in hemorrhage patients develop a pale color." Later in the same book, there are two brothers who bleed from the rectum, and they too become pale.

A man turns cold and white in death. And at the Apocalypse, at the end of time, Death rides a pale horse.

A paleface is half a man. Once the term was used to contrast a European in America from a so-called red man. Later, a paleface signified a weakling. The ever-volatile Wyndham Lewis, in his extended essay *Paleface: The Philosophy of the "Melting-Pot"* (1929), blasts multiculturalism as a white man's inferiority complex, an effete surrender of virile European cultural vigor. In his essay "Paleface and Redskin" (1939), the critic Philip Rahv, cofounder of the *Partisan Review*, uses the terms to contrast indoor, sensitive, patrician esthetes with outdoors, roughshod, plebeian lowbrows. Henry James is a paleface, Walt Whitman a redskin. The paleface too may indicate excessive cerebralism, contrasted with soulfulness, as in the famous anecdote in which the Pueblo chief Ochwiay Biano tells Jung that the problem with white men is that they think with their heads, while the Pueblo think with their hearts. And then there is the 1948 movie *The Paleface*, in which Bob Hope plays a bumbling and cowardly dentist in the Wild West.

If every word forms a pair with its opposite, or with a set of potential opposites, what stands opposite to pale cheeks? First is blushing: the modest maiden's cheeks turn red. In *Romeo and Juliet*, the heroine on the balcony professes girlish innocence:

> Thou knowest the mask of night is on my face,
> Else would a maiden blush bepaint my cheek.

Whether she blushes unseen, hidden by night, or instead does not blush at all, is left for the auditor to decide.

The cheeks redden too in arousal, whether amorous or otherwise. A few moments after the balcony scene, Juliet's nurse tells her charge of the assignation in Friar Lawrence's cell and comments on a change she observes: "Now comes the wanton blood up in your cheeks." Chaucer's Wife of Bath, that archetypal woman of too many husbands, is constitutionally red-faced:

> Bold was hir face, and fair, and reed of hewe.
> She was a worthy womman al hir lyve:
> Housbondes at chirche dore she hadde fyve

Do authors and authorities depict feminine arousal as predominantly sexual?

So too might be a man's, but masculine reddening is anger, sturdiness, readiness for fight. The red-cheeked man is ruddy and sanguinary. Esau, firstborn son of Isaac, is red and hairy, a man of the field. Mars is red—the planet Mars is red, the color attribute of the god Mars is red, his element is iron.

Or the red-cheeked man might be besotted. Habitual tippling causes the capillaries of the face and nose to dilate, imparting a chronic redness. Chaucer describes his Franklin thus:

> Of his complexioun he was sangwyn.
> Wel loved he by the morwe a sop in wyn.

The porter in *Macbeth* has been carousing and reports, famously, that "drink, sir, is a great provoker of three things . . . nose-painting, sleep, and urine." W. C. Fields played the character of the red-nosed sottish scallywag, though the actor's bulbous proboscis resulted from rosacea, a chronic inflammation of the skin, not from drink.

The face flushes in triumph and conquest, the male's province again.

But—the face turns red in fever.

The terms negotiate one with another, the words shift. "Florid," in the dictionary, is a healthy, rosy hue; but in common usage, an overly red face is *florid with rage, florid with drink.* The sanguinary temperament of medieval physiology, in which blood predominated over the other three humors, could be cheerful, courageous, amiable, or amorous.

Pallor is the white where color once was, an unnatural and fearful sucked-out, bleached-out absence, an exsanguination.

Are they polar opposites, pale *contra* red, or a continuum? Midway between too pale and too red, a pleasant pink hue signals health and forthrightness. In Melville's *Billy Budd*, "The Shipmaster was one of those worthy mortals found in every vocation, even the humbler ones—the sort of person whom everybody agrees in calling 'a respectable man.' . . . For the rest, he was fifty or thereabouts, a little inclined to corpulence, a prepossessing face, unwhiskered, and of an agreeable color—a rather full face, humanely intelligent in expression." And later in the same tale we read the following contrast between the protagonist and the villain: "But the form of Billy Budd was heroic; and if his face was without the intellectual look of the pallid Claggart's, not the less was it lit, like his, from within, though from a different source. The bonfire in his heart made luminous the rose-tan in his cheek."

For Ovid, to cite one of many sources, the young woman's rosy complexion demonstrates her vitality, though complexion and vitality both shall fade with age. François Villon, the melancholic, brawling, scholar-thief-poet of fifteenth-century Paris, forecasts the decrepitude of a woman who has spurned him by picturing her "ugly, without color." For Ovid, again, cosmetics can supplant what Nature has not bestowed or Time has taken away. But too much rouge indicates venery, lust, the painted lady, the scarlet woman, the harlot.

One can thus imagine a spectrum, from pale to plethoric:

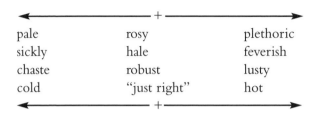

pale	rosy	plethoric
sickly	hale	feverish
chaste	robust	lusty
cold	"just right"	hot

Villon professes to know both sides:

> Prince, I know all in sum
> I know the colored and the pale
> I know Death who consumes all
> I know everything except myself.

And the bride in the *Song of Songs* would have it both ways: "My beloved is white and ruddy, the chiefest among ten thousand."

3. The Malice Sickle

THE AMBULANCE BRINGS A SIX-YEAR-OLD BOY TO THE emergency department. Aaron has terrible pain in his knee. He has had this pain before; the nurses and doctors all know him. They know him well, they say. He has sickle-cell anemia.

The boy grows to be a man. Aaron is a small, thin man. He comes to the hospital every few months, and perhaps he goes to other hospitals in the interim. Every time it is the same. The doctors give him medicine, pain medicine, powerful medicine—morphine and its close congeners hydromorphone, oxycodone, meperidine—or perhaps it is not so strong as the doctors say, for they still the pain, assuredly, briefly, the pain recedes but always it returns.

Aaron's limbs are thin. They carry little muscle and little fat. The joints seem large, the elbows and knees, for young men's joints know but one size. The fat man's joints disappear into the adjacent flesh, the emaciated man's joints stand out in harsh contrast to the lean long bones they link. Aaron has sickle-cell, Aaron is sickly, he never has exercised, has never borne for long his skinny body's weight, though it weighs him down. Aaron has not known running, or has long forgotten it; what Aaron knows and remembers is pain, and a brief forgetting when the pain is briefly gone.

Sickle-cell anemia is a disease of hemoglobin, the oxygen-carrying molecule of the red blood cell. The DNA in a person with sickle-cell anemia has a single change (compared with the rest of us) that codes for a single molecular alteration that produces a radically different hemoglobin. This changed hemoglobin changes its shape, under certain circumstances, from the usual flexible disk into an inflexible, crescent-shaped cell, the sickle cell. These rigid sickled cells are unable to pass through the tiny capillaries and therefore obstruct them. The result of blocked capillaries is severe, unremitting pain in the flesh and bone. This is the sickle crisis. Picture tying a tight belt around your leg and leaving it there, perhaps a long time. The leg hurts, a little and then a lot, the leg begins to die a little, and so the sickle patient dies a little, every time, from early childhood on.

Sickle-cell anemia occurs most often in people of African ancestry, especially those from a broad band on each side of the equator. It also occurs, although less famously, in people whose origins stem from southern Europe, the Near East, India, and Southeast Asia. In the United States, sickle cell is a disease of African Americans, or so it is known. One forms an image of a poor black child of the city, an Aaron, who comes to the hospital and returns and returns.

How could God permit such a disease, which torments poor children? It turns out that only people with two abnormal genes are so afflicted. The person with one abnormal gene, who is said to have sickle trait, is not only well but also partially protected against a major scourge of the tropical world, malaria. Thus, God or Nature tortures the few so that the many may resist malaria. In the language of Darwinian biology, to be a sickle carrier conveys a selective reproductive advantage, resistance to malaria, which perpetuates the (selfish) gene even at the cost of sacrificing the few to the tortures of sickle-cell disease.

American and European physicians define people with sickle trait as healthy "carriers" who bear no ill effect from their genetic status. The picture looks different in Senegal, where such persons often feel that sickle trait makes them sick. Senegalese patients and their physicians frequently attribute symptoms to sickle trait that mainstream medicine assigns to other causes, especially to psychological and social stress. The sickle label thus reifies the patient's distress and the doctor's attempt to name otherwise uncategorized symptoms. Senegalese patients, meanwhile, may take affront that a bioscientific doctor rejects their understanding of their own suffering.

From a molecular perspective, the disease is fascinating. The first description in the medical literature dates to 1910, although the discovery properly belongs less to the author, James B. Herrick, than to his intern, Ernest Irons. (Herrick, by the way, became famous; Irons remains nearly unknown.) A generation later, sickle-cell anemia was the first molecular disease, the first to be identified as arising from a changed molecule. Words fall short, for what shall we call this altered gene? "Abnormal," "mutated," "defective," these imply pejorative contrast with the normal and, incidentally, "white" version. "Variant" errs on the opposite side, too neutral, avoiding judgment but missing the pain. Fascinating, too, is the concept that carriers bore evolutionary advantage, for now we look for such benefit whenever we meet a genetic disease. Might hemochromatosis, which causes the body to overabsorb iron, bring benefit to peoples whose diets were low in iron? Might Down syndrome (Trisomy 21) be a genetic experiment that trades intelligence for kindness?

The scientists are fascinated. The doctors are discouraged. For they have little to offer Aaron. They cannot cure him, they can barely treat him, and only in the crudest way, pain meds, morphine and such, the gentle hammer. Aaron meets suspicion, for none can confirm his pain, they have only his testimony, he says he is in pain, we believe or we do not, we err at our peril, and his. To deny pain relief to a suffering patient violates every decent medical principle. But to give pain medications, opiates, to a malingerer is to support the unwanted behavior and to create an unending cycle of drugs and habit. To prescribe to an abuser (how defined?), or even to a legitimate user with higher than ordinary dosing, might subject the physician to censure or even criminal prosecution. How shall we know? Pain is the subjective experience of suffering, Aaron reports that he is suffering, and who shall contradict him?

The medical mind conceives a notion of pain medicine *just enough*, the dose that provides analgesia without excessive sedation. For most incidents of pain, the doctor can predict the effective dose. A broken leg should warrant about ten milligrams of morphine. Less would be insufficient, the pain would not abate. More would be excessive, the patient would be stuporous. In between, the patient is comfortable but alert. And yet this happy medium is hard to find in patients with sickle cell, they writhe in anguish one moment and sleep in torpor the next. The doctor is frustrated, peeved, angry, the recipe didn't work, and who is to blame—the doctor, the patient, the disease?

Sickle defies clinical empathy, the doctor mistrusts the patient's report of pain, the doctor withholds, the doctor does not engage. Sickle happens to someone else, someone unlike myself, a black someone, his pain is not mine. The patient too mistrusts the doctor, why won't he treat my pain, why does he disbelieve?

The body constantly pained learns to be in pain. No pain medication ever suffices for the brain whose circuits expect pain, when every neurological signal sounds an alarm of unremitting pain.

Some 80,000 Americans are thought to have the disease, one in every 4,000 of us. It results in 750,000 hospitalizations per year. The cost of these hospitalizations comes to some $475 million, not to speak of outpatient costs, the drugs and tests and doctors' visits, and who shall quantify the human costs? Not every patient with sickle-cell disease is Aaron. Some live quite differently, some live and work and face their disease as one with asthma might, or diabetes—a condition to manage. But these are not the patients whom the doctors come to know, and least of all the doctors in the hospital, and theirs is not the drama.

The disease is named "sickle-cell anemia." *Sickle*—the cell is a sickle, but why not a crescent, a comma, a banana? The sickle is an ancient tool, the instrument of reaping, the instrument of death, the grim reaper. In tarot, the Death card of the major arcana portrays a skeleton bearing a sickle. With a flint or adamantine sickle Kronos castrates his father, Uranos, and indeed the sickle patient rarely bears children, rarely bears the full adult burdens of procreation and work, rarely reaps but is himself reaped and all too early reaped— or maybe not too soon, for what is his life of awful recurring pain, or who is to say it should be lived or no? The cruel irony here is that the Aarons are prone to priapism, a painful erection that will not go away. The Greek Kronos corresponds to the Roman Saturn, whose astrological and later astronomical symbol is said to represent an inverted sickle. Saturn is the dour deity, he presides over death and melancholy, the artist some say lives under the sign of Saturn.

Cell—the disease is a problem of the cell, the "*cellula*," as the first microscopists named those hitherto invisible biological units, a little room, a monk's chamber, a prison cell, a lonely nook, a cell. The famed diseases have ancient names, pneumonia, pleurisy, carcinoma, apoplexy, catarrh, how few are named for a cell.

Anemia—the disease is a deficiency of blood, though the

patient knows pain, not pallor, not breathlessness. To call the disease anemia gives voice to the microscope but not to the pain, the doctor knows the microscope, the patient knows the pain, they contest the name, they contest the dose of pain medication.

They contest, too, the day of hospital discharge. An illness episode, a drama, has a beginning, a middle, and an end. The modern hospital would admit only those patients too ill to survive at home, or those who need some hospital-based procedure—an operation, for example. As soon as these "acute" services are no longer needed, the patient must go home. The pneumonia is resolving, the heart attack has stabilized, the surgery is over, the hospitalization draws to a close, the patient goes home. But what of a disease that has no end? The sickle patient is admitted for treatments, injections of narcotics, that cannot be given at home, but when is he well enough to go home? The doctor, accustomed to short and well-defined illness episodes, says *now* or *soon*. The sickle patient, accustomed to long and ill-defined illness episodes, says *no*, or *not yet*, or maybe nothing at all, or maybe a threatened *never*. The hospital pressures the doctor, Aaron's length of stay is growing long. The doctor tries to coax Aaron, and Aaron responds in his only language, pain, and with his only resistance, no, not yet.

We live in the age of the gene, also in the age of calculations and probabilities, of calculated risks, of risk-benefit ratios, of estimated returns on investments. If two sickle carriers intend a family, the likelihood is twenty-five percent that any given child will have sickle disease, fifty percent that he will be a sickle carrier, and twenty-five percent that he will bear no sickle hemoglobin at all. In the first instance his life will likely be one of recurrent pain and early death; in the second, an ordinary life like that of his parents; in the third, an ordinary life without genetic baggage, the chain has been stopped, the witch is dead. What shall a parent do? Contemporary Medicine would test the parents, a simple blood test, and if both are carriers would test the fetus, a much more complicated affair; and if the fetus has sickle-cell disease, would consider abortion. Better not to exist than to live a life of sickle pain. One still hears doctors complain at times, they are tired, they have admitted Aarons before, sickle, they say, is a disease of inadequate genetic counseling. Aaron should not be.

Viewed from the patient's perspective, antenatal testing for sickle-cell disease is more nuanced. For example, the medical anthropologist Duana Fullwiley found that Senegalese physicians felt that their patients would not accept antenatal testing for sickle cell anemia, positing such barriers as "tradition," "the need of Africans to bear children," and Muslim belief. However, when asked in their own homes, most sickle-cell patients and family members said that they would welcome antenatal testing, and a third said that they would abort an affected fetus. Fullwiley also found that the people she interviewed associated sickle-cell disease not with genetics in general but with consanguineous marriage in specific, as people in Senegal most commonly wed relatives in marriages arranged by the extended family. For some women, premarital testing for sickle trait might afford them the otherwise impossible prerogative to refuse an unwanted cousin or uncle as husband.

The rhetoric of Medicine speaks of diseases that spread. The immediate subject is infectious disease, contagion. Tuberculosis spreads when one person transmits it to another, and so does syphilis, and so does the common cold. But medical talk of sickle-cell disease also spoke of spreading, as if the parent infects or contaminates the child, as if the black parent were a carrier, a secret bearer of disease, as if the parent corrupts the child and the genetic stock of all society.

Aaron is no dummy, even if he is narcotized half the time, he intuits their weary sentiment, they wish that he were not. The doctors take an oath, they relieve suffering, they preserve life, but not for me, they would that I were not. Certainly not here, in their hospital, or at least not on their shift.

One speaks of sickle crisis. This is the last remnant, the ultimate vestige of an ancient Hippocratic concept, the crisis, to each disease its climax, the critical day, the point at which it turns to recovery or to death, from "*krinein*," to decide. The awful pain is termed a crisis, and yet the sickle patient knows no crisis, no climax, no turning point, and no decision, only recurrent catastrophe.

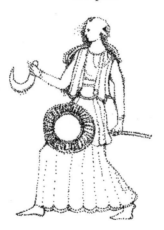

The slaying of Orpheus

II. DIAGNOSIS /
WHAT'S WRONG

The physician, whether of this century or some other, hears the patient's story and relates it to a disease framework. This is an act of translation, therefore an act of transformation and distortion, seizing the patient's tale and making it the doctor's own. This arrogation, sometimes gentle, sometimes violent, provides the basis for clinical action. The doctor, meanwhile, knows somewhere, or ought to know, that bella donna *and* beautiful lady *are not the same, and neither are* weakness *and* anemia.

4. The Green Sicknesse

THE POET SAPPHO, AMONG THE GREATEST WHO EVER LIVED, writes of a girl who espies her beloved:

> and sweat pours down me
> fear seizes me
> I am paler than new grass
> and would nearly die

The Greek word translated as "paler than new grass" is *chlōrotera*, from *chlōros*, "green" or "pale." *Chlōros* gives us chlorophyll, the green pigment of plants, and chlorine, the pale green gas. The related *chloē* is a fresh shoot, a young leaf or blade of grass, and gives us the girl's name.

Lady Macbeth accuses her husband of cowardice:

> Was the hope drunk
> Wherein you dressed yourself? Hath it slept since?
> And wakes it now to look so green and pale
> At what it did so freely?

What do the poets mean by green? I have never seen a person green. The green man, yes, the green man whose effigy stood before an English pub, the nature man, Sir Gawain and the Green Knight, Papageno, the Jolly Green Giant, all green and wild, all fictive. But if a girl or man does not turn literally green, whence comes this conceit?

In 1554, the Swiss-born physician Johannes Lange defines a new disease. Writing in the form of a letter—that genre of proto-essay, disguised in personal terms, meant for posterity—to a friend whose daughter is ailing, the Leipzig professor notes:

> the qualities of her face, which in the past year was distinguished by rosiness of cheeks and redness of lips, is some how as if exsanguinated, sadly paled, the heart trembles with every movement of her body, and the arteries of her temples pulsate, & she is seized with dyspnoea in dancing or climbing the stairs, her stomach loathes food and particularly meat, & the legs, especially at the ankles, become edematous at night.

He calls this condition the "Disease of Virgins." He perceives the young woman's pallor, her rapid heart rate, and shortness of breath, all symptoms of what a modern would call anemia. He furthermore relates her state to a deficiency of blood, "as if exsanguinated." He notes that she avoids food, which a modern might relate to anorexia nervosa, more a cause than a result of anemia. He compares it to "white fever, or pale face & the fever of love," and he goes on to assert that the cause is a blockage in the internal flow of menstrual blood, which contaminates the vital organs. The cure is marriage, and specifically, coition.

Later authors call Lange's treatise the first clinical description of the disease chlorosis, or the green sickness—though the Swiss physician used neither term. By the late sixteenth century, English authors speak abundantly of the green sickness. Thus Robert Greene's *Mamillia* (1583): "that his daughter being at the age of twentie yeeres, would either fall into the green sicknes for want of a husband, or els if she scaped that disease, incurre a farther inconvenience." Shakespeare, a contemporary, has Falstaff complain about the

Duke of Lancaster, the sober brother of Hal the Prince, who has rebuked him:

> There's never none of these demure boys come to any proof, for thin drink doth so over-cool their blood, and making many fish-meals, that they fall into a kind of male green sickness, and then when they marry, they get wenches.

That is, the disease has already been well established as properly belonging to women, and if Lancaster is so afflicted, he is so pusillanimous as to beget only daughters.

In 1619, students of the recently deceased French physician Jean Varandal, professor of medicine at Montpellier, publish a book on the diseases of women that summarizes his teachings and introduces the term "chlorosis" for the first time.

> Which the common people call pale or fetid colors, white icterus, amatory fever, or the disease of virgins, but we, from Hippocrates, call chlorosis, because it is a kind of cachexia accompanied by a certain abnormal white or greenish color.

The Montpellier professor claims to find the term in a newly discovered text attributed to Hippocrates, *On the Diseases of Young Women*—although the word is not found in the Greek original.

The celebrated seventeenth-century English physician Thomas Sydenham describes the green sickness in terms closely observed and empiric—or seemingly so. "The face and body lose colour, the face also swells; so do the eyelids and ankles. The body feels heavy; there is a tension and lassitude in the legs and feet, dyspnoea, palpitation of the heart, headache, febrile pulse, somnolence, pica, and suppression of the menses." Pica refers to eating dirt and clay, of which more later. Pallor, here, but nothing green in the green sickness. The loss of menses echoes the "Disease of Virgins" and their blocked internal menstrual arrangements. Indeed, Sydenham considers chlorosis to be a species of hysteria, resulting from a weakening of spirit, "a faulty disposition of the animal spirits," and consequently an accumulation of putrid humors. The treatment is therefore restoration and fortification of the blood, the conveyor of spirit. For this, he prescribes bleeding (to remove contaminants) followed by iron preparations of various sorts. The latter could come in the form of a chalybeate, an iron-rich mineral water, as well as steel filings, iron ore, or a syrup of these suspended in wine. This diagnosis and plan sounds remarkably close to the modern conception of iron-deficiency anemia—until one considers that Sydenham touts iron not for its mineral characteristics but rather for its ancient humoral and even alchemical properties. His concept of blood as the conveyor of spirit recapitulates late medieval views—for example, those of the great thirteenth-century physician Arnauld of Villanova—more than it anticipates modern ones.

From the sixteenth through the nineteenth centuries, the green sickness / chlorosis forms a complex of symptoms and observations, occurring almost always in adolescent and young women: pallor, debility, rapid heart rate, breathlessness, digestive irregularities, menstrual disorders, difficulties in love. The cure is usually sex. Or, in the comic prescription of Montesquieu (1721):

> *A cure for chlorosis, vulgarly called the green-sickness, or hot fit of love.* Take four plates from Aretinus; take of Thomas Sanchez' work on Marriage, two leaves. Infuse them in five pounds of common water, and you will have a pleasant aperient.

His joke is to combine Aretino's naughty books with a Jesuit priest's manual on conjugal relations. An aperient is a laxative.

Doctor Johnson's *Dictionary* (1755) provides no entry for "anemia" or "anaemia" but does define "chlorosis," calling it simply "the green-sickness." The entry for "green" gives two definitions, the first the color, the second as follows: "Pale; sickly; from whence we call the maid's disease the green sickness, or chlorosis, Like it is Sappho's χλωροτέρα."

The green sickness became a European phenomenon. The French called it *pâles couleurs*, pale colors, or *mal d'amour*, love sickness. The Germans called it *Bleichsucht*, pale longing.

That chlorosis was a multifaceted illness of young women, all agreed. What these facets were was a matter of controversy. Included in all definitions were notions of pallor, weakness, fragility, and oversensitivity. For Baudelaire, chlorosis is, like pallor, an indoor phenomenon; its enemy, in his poem "Le Soleil," is the sun. Additional overtones veered towards sexual and menstrual dysfunction. The cause was unknown. Some authorities invoked a weakness of the blood, others uneven stages of physiologic development, others an undersized heart, others deficient diet, others a nervous disorder, others hysteria. But authors are nearly unanimous on one strange point: *the girls looked green*. Physicians, especially, spoke of a greenish hue that was readily apparent to the discerning clinical eye. They wrote so often of the disease in nineteenth-century Britain and America that it seemed nearly an epidemic.

But just about that time, toward the turn of the last century, a new idea stepped forth: chlorosis is iron-deficiency anemia. It was a simple explanation, one fully consonant with the growing notion that health and disease consisted primarily in biomechanical function and malfunction. Girls were simply not obtaining enough iron in their diets, they were not eating enough meat. And lo and behold—the green sickness disappears. By the early twentieth century, physicians remark that chlorosis has become extinct.

Truly extinct? Céline, in his 1931 novel *Guignol's Band*, writes of "Berthe, the skinny green-looking one." The scene is a brothel, the narrator a Frenchman in the London underworld during the First World War. The author is a physician.

And even today, chlorosis remains a term in the alternative practices of homeopathy, naturopathy, and related fields. A search on Google (April 2007) yields some 1,650,000 "hits"; on Amazon.com, some 2,260. (Admittedly, many of these refer to plant diseases of the same name—though one might speculate how and why these were so named.)

In an informal poll of twenty-first-century hematologists at a major academic medical center, none had heard of chlorosis or the green sickness. And one more point: all had seen iron-deficiency anemia, but *none had ever seen the patient appear green*. Something isn't adding up. One comes to a bothersome question: *Did the girls with the green sickness ever look green?*

In the standard dictionary of classical Greek, *chlōros* bears three main senses:

I.   *greenish-yellow* (like young grass or leaves), *pale-green, light-green, green, grassy.*

II. generally, *pale, pallid, bleached*

III. without regard to colour, *green*, i.e., *fresh*   2. metaph. *fresh, living.*

The root is *chloē*, "*the first shoot of plants* in spring, *the green blade of corn or grass*."

The Hippocratic medical texts of the fifth and fourth centuries BCE use *chlōros* in all these senses. Thus, the book *Prognostic* describes the famous Hippocratic facies, the appearance of a man approaching death. The color of the face is "*chlōron e melan*," *chlōros* or black. Later, the same book says that it is a bad sign if the stools are "very fluid, or white, or exceedingly green [*chlōron*] or frothy." It is also an unfavorable sign if the sputum is *chlōron*, or if the stool discharges pus that is *chlōron* or livid. Children suffer seizures if their color, during fever, becomes *chlōron*, livid, or red. Here, the standard English translator renders *chlōron* variously as pale, yellow, exceedingly green, or light green, depending on context and on his own interpretation of circumstances.

Also in cough, green means bad. The man with green sputum wants an antibiotic, the man with clear sputum is content without, though both most likely have a simple cold.

In the world of color symbolism, green is the color of Venus the planet, Venus the goddess, love, gladness, venery. In contrast, the color of Mars is red, his metal is iron, iron is red; this is the probable basis of Sydenham's prescription of iron to treat the green sickness. Iron bolsters the martial aspect and vivifies the spirit.

Green is not only a color but also a field of associations. Green is youthful, inexperienced, unschooled, innocent, untamed—a green recruit, a green goose. Green is also vigorous, lusty, and green is also unripe, unready. Green too is blooming, verdant. Small wonder that in England, until the time of Elizabeth I, wedding dresses were green. What better word, what better color, for the complicated dilemma of young womanhood, ready and unready. (And to whom, and for whom? The men who father them, the others who court them, or would court them, the men who wed them, the physicians who hear their symptoms or hear others tell their symptoms and try to fit them into a comprehensible pattern, she seems somehow unwell, what might it be, perhaps she has the green sickness, perhaps she looks green.

Approaching the Athenian Acropolis, near the sanctuary of the healing god Asklepios, there stood a shrine to Demeter Chloe, the harvest goddess in her green avatar, mother as maiden.

Green is the opposite color to red. A pale or anemic cheek is notable for its lack of redness, it is un-red or anti-red. Look at the sun and then a blank white field and you will see a violet disk, the color opposite of the sun's yellow; look at a blank white face, where you expect to see red, and you might well see green. Never mind that a blank white field and a blank white face are not the same thing.

The girl's green hue is thus a projection of the beholder, based on mistaken Greek when the language had first arrived in northern Europe, based on mistaken readings of a Hippocratic text when it too had newly arrived, based on centuries of associations and echoes of green and all its meanings. It was a whisper-down-the-lane phenomenon, of a type all too familiar in medicine. The great Galen asserted that the liver has four lobes. He probably came to this conclusion by dissecting Barbary apes, for the human liver has no such lobes; but centuries of physicians repeated the four-lobed-liver error and obliged their students to recite the same wrong answer.

People fall ill. How they (and the rest of us) understand their feelings of unwellness is remarkably complex, depending not only on the immediate sensation of pain or other discomfort but on the highly mediated effects of symptom configuration, social norms, expectations of health and disease, personal experience, and naming. Every culture and subculture has its framework for comprehending health and disease, its overarching theories of medicine, and every illness episode is translated into the terms of this great (even if unwritten) book of diseases. How well the physician's disease matches the patient's illness is a source of considerable friction. The shoe may not fit—if it doesn't, it rubs and raises blisters.

A modern physician sees a teenager who tires easily; she looks pale, her heart is rapid. If she was fine yesterday, she might just be in love. If the condition has persisted, she might still be in love, but she probably has anemia. A blood test will solve the latter puzzle in a day—though certainly not the former. That, in any event, is not the province of the modern physician. Anemia is the proper object of his attention, not love.

The physician of a century or two ago, seeing the same girl, would have no concept of anemia but would think quickly of chlorosis. Does she have the other symptoms of that diagnostic constellation? Are her evacuations irregular —why, yes, they are a bit, and whose are not in that north European regimen of sausage and potatoes, few vegetables and fewer fruits (deemed dangerous), little exercise? Are her menses irregular—why, yes, but how many teenagers have completely regular menses? And anyway how unpleasant a topic, shall we broach it only in euphemism and indirection. Are her ankles swollen, perhaps not, perhaps a little towards the end of the day (and whose would not be in a corset?)? Does she look green? Perhaps she does.

The expectations that society and family place on the patient often influence the sense of what is normal and abnormal, or right and wrong. Was the diagnosis, chlorosis, a means of diseasifying the social and psychological conditions of a young woman? Was she too idle, or too active, or too sexual, or too unsexual, too menstrual, too unmenstrual, or did she eat too little, or too much? Was she too urban, too educated, too blonde, too confined, too free?

And then there was the name. The pale breathless girl was green, fresh, innocent, unripe, inexperienced but *on the brink of experience*—Venus the morning star, Venus the evening star, a creature of Venus, under the sign of Venus, venereal.

Why did chlorosis disappear? Some say that girls nowadays are simply better fed; others that the expression of adolescent stress morphed into other forms, anorexia, for example, or depression; and others that the artificial construction simply fell down. In any event, the metaphor and its projection no longer served, the chain of whispers was broken, the emperor's new green clothes. And yet one central feature of the diagnosis persists, from the green sickness to iron-deficiency anemia: to know or misknow the adolescent girl through her nascent sexuality, to know her primarily as a being becoming sexual, attributed to blocked menses five hundred years ago, to flowing menses (and its attendant iron loss) today. How close the words, languish, languid, languor.

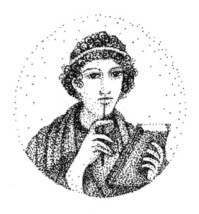

The chlorotic, the girl looks green—well, I don't see it yet, but I am just a student, my teacher my master assures me that it is so, and maybe she does look a little green, certainly piqued, attractive, in fact, amorous, perhaps, to be embraced, not to be embraced, for me, not for me.

5. Anemia's Old Tale

IN *THE ILIAD*, THE HERO DIOMEDES WOUNDS THE GODDESS
Aphrodite, and

> blood flowed from the immortal goddess,
> ichor, which flows through the blessed gods,
> for they neither eat grain nor drink flashing wine,
> and therefore are bloodless and are called deathless.

The word here rendered as "bloodless" is *anhaimones*,
an + haimon, no blood. Blood is the essence of life but also
of mortality, and through the veins of the immortals flows
the fluid ichor, a divine counterpart to mortal blood.

The word "anemia," which appears here for the first
time, is very far from the later concept of a deficiency of
blood. From a medical perspective, the oldest concept was
not anemia but pallor. The so-called Hippocratic facies, the
appearance of a man nearing death, is pale—indicating, in
modern terms, reduced blood flow to the face. As the concept of pallor becomes more medicalized, physicians recognize a condition of skin paleness throughout the body. The
text *Epidemics* describes an outbreak of fever and cough,
accompanied by what might be translated "whitishness" or
"near whiteness." And in the disease called White Phlegm
(*phlegma leukon*):

the patient's skin appears whiter because his blood, in consequence of the large amount of phlegm, becomes more watery than normal, so that the usual healthy color is no longer present in it to the degree that it was before; thus, patients appear whiter and the disease is called white phlegm.

Most importantly, the author attributes pallor to a condition of the blood—perhaps the first time in Western medicine that this relation is documented. Watery blood—this is very near the modern concept of anemia, a deficiency of the cellular elements that give blood its color and thickness.

Aristotle seems to allude to watery blood when writing of animals. "If the blood get exceedingly liquid, animals fall sick; for the blood then turns into something like ichor, or a liquid so thin that it at times has been known to exude through the pores like sweat." Aristotle has adopted the term ichor to mean not the vital, insubstantial fluid of the gods but something more resembling what we would call the lymph, the clear fluid of the lymphatic system. Lymph *can* exude through the skin when a body part is very swollen, as might occur in severe disease of the heart, liver, or kidneys. Blood would so exude rarely or never.

Curious: although many patients bleed in the Hippocratic texts, or are bled, they are not described as pale. Thus, the Greek physicians, in the main, seem to associate pallor with a blood deficiency of some type but not blood loss. Similarly, *The Iliad* describes scores of gruesome battlefield deaths, but none of the falling warriors becomes wan as his arms clatter about him.

The Roman medical tradition had little to say of pallor and nothing of anemia, concerned more with systematizing and codifying Greek medical theory than with clinical observation or vatic dream. One might say, a bit unkindly but not unjustly, that Roman medicine resembles Greek as

do the triumphs of their respective architectures, the aque-
duct contrasted with the Temple of Poseidon at Sounion.

In the Ayurvedic tradition of India, pallor is denoted by
the Sanskrit term *pándu*. The classic *Suśruta Samhitā*, compiled
in the first century CE of materials developed in the preceding five hundred years or more, groups *pāndu* together with
jaundice, known as *kāmalā*. (Of note, the Hippocratic and
Roman traditions also group together pallor and jaundice,
two overt species of skin discoloration.) These occur "from
vitiation of the blood from imbalance of the humours in
people who indulge in excessive sexual intercourse and
intake of sour and pungent substances, salts, wine, earth, and
who sleep by day." The three Ayurvedic humors are *vāta*
(wind/breath/air), *pitta* (bile/fire), and *kapha* (phlegm/mucus
/water). When *pāndu* affects *kapha*, the body (and its secre-
tions) are white. The treatments are many, including iron,
which is especially recommended for severe pallor. Thus, in
general terms, we have the concept of sick blood, associated
with pallor, that can be treated with iron. This idea, although
embedded in multiple matters of a very different sort, predates the Euro-American equivalent by more than fifteen
hundred years.

Pallor also occurs if a patient is bled excessively, accompanied by "headache, disturbed vision fits, paralysis, shortness
of breath." Here too the Indian physicians articulate a point
on which the Greek and Roman authors remain silent.

During the European Middle Ages, the most advanced
medicine and science of the Western world belonged to the
realms of Islam, stretching from southern Asia and northern
India across Persia, Asia Minor, the Middle East, and North
Africa to Spain. Its greatest exponent was Abū Alī al-Husayn
ibn Abd Allāh ibn Sīnā (980–1037), known to Europe as
Avicenna. His *Canon of Medicine*, the foremost medical textbook of many centuries, conceived of pallor both as a con-

dition of the blood and as a particular configuration of the four humors. For Ibn Sīnā, "Pallor indicates a cold temperament and the accompanying feature is lack of blood. Yellowish color indicates a hot temperament which is accompanied by lack of blood, and increase of bilious humor. Ruddiness indicates a hot temperament with abundance of blood, sanguine or bilious temperament. Sub-ruddiness indicates a hot temperament with dominance of bilious humor. Occasionally it denotes lack of blood, provided there is no bilious humor present in the blood as is the case in convalescence." The Persian master, situated midway between the Roman and Indian worlds, thus melds their two ideas of pallor, Galenic systematizing and Ayurvedic empiricism.

If Avicenna ruled medical thinking for half a millennium, his most provocatory challenge came from the Swiss-born physician Philippus Aureolus Theophrastus Bombastus von Hohenheim (1492–1541), known as Paracelsus. Whether he chose this appellation himself or received it from another hand, and whether it refers to claiming a position "beyond Celsus" (the Roman encyclopedist and medical authority) or to something else, is lost to myth. Paracelsus, a contemporary of Dürer, Luther, Erasmus (whom he treated), and George Faust, the prototype of the legend, was an itinerant and iconoclastic figure. In 1527, newly appointed as professor at Basel, he publicly burned the works of Avicenna and Galen on the steps of the university—or so it was said. His personal motto, like an invented blazon on a coat of arms, reads "I am different, let this not upset you."

He grew up in the mining country of the Tyrol, that ancient mountainous region now divided among Switzerland, Germany, Austria, and Italy. There he learned firsthand the earthy, underground, sooty, grimy qualities of minerals, their tactile and olfactory properties, the digging and crushing and smelting of ore, the fiery foundry and forge, also the injuries and sicknesses of miners. Some have credited his treatise *On the Miners' Sickness and Other Miners' Diseases* (1567) as the earliest work devoted to occupational medicine. Paracelsus became the first European to champion the use of minerals in the treatment of disease, for the main pharmacologic approach since the Greeks had been to prescribe herbs. Most famous was his use of mercury for the treatment of syphilis, a disease that exploded across the Old World shortly after the discovery of the New. Mercury worked pretty well, and although its toxicities could be terrible, it remained the mainstay of therapy until the twentieth century.

Paracelsus also prescribed compounds of arsenic, gold, copper—and iron, probably the first European doctor to do so. Medicine was becoming chemical.

In the 1660s, a thirty-something Dutch linen draper named Antonie van Leeuwenhoek developed the peculiar hobby of grinding lenses and looking at tiny objects under magnification. Among the subjects of his unusual and remarkably sharp-sighted regard were the microscopic "animalcules" that were later known as bacteria and protozoa. In 1684, he turned his attention to the blood and reported the presence of tiny globules. These became known as the red corpuscles, later called red blood cells, or erythrocytes. In the ensuing decades, microscopists began not only to observe the red cells more closely but also to consider them the essential element of blood. (Although their instruments were entirely new, the theoretical underpinning was ancient. Asclepiades, in the first century BCE, had applied the atomism of Democritus to medicine and argued that health and disease consisted in the balance of minute solid particles, or corpuscles. And Leeuwenhoek's contemporary Robert Boyle, "the father of chemistry," was arguing that all natural phenomena could be explained by the position and motion of corpuscles. (Boyle, it may be added, was another of the great early scientists who was also fascinated by alchemy.)

Sometimes the red corpuscles seemed pale under the microscope, and this occurred in patients who seemed pale. Pallor was newly seen as a problem of the red blood cells. Thus Albrecht von Haller (1708–77), one of the great early experimentalists: "Hemorrhage produces degeneration of the blood which is normally red and dense and which becomes pale and serous."

The next challenge was to count the corpuscles, and the nineteenth century invented the apparatuses for doing so. A new concept arises, that blood deficiency is a matter of *too few* red cells. To commemorate the occasion, English and French create a new word, anaemia, anemia, *anémie*. The *Oxford English Dictionary*'s earliest citation is from 1836. The word is Greek. The word, in its medical usage, is fake Greek. Whether the modern creators of the term copped it from the Homeric Greek, or instead coined it anew, I have never learned. Anemia is *a* + *haema*, no + blood. Anemia is the privation of blood. Anemia is bloodless, without blood, having no blood. The medical word signifies loss, not divinity. It is an invention of modern Europeans, sanctifying their idea with a sham lineage, a phony coat of arms. The Germans, following their own Teutonic path, serve the same purpose to different effect with *Blutarmut*, blood poverty.

By the time a generation passes, the red blood count is considered the most accurate way to diagnose anemia.

See what has happened here. The original issue was pallor. Although there were some early hints relating pallor to a deficiency of the blood, millennia were to pass before medicine made this connection firmly. The crucial modern step was to count the red blood cells. From this point onward, the *count* is the essential hematologic act. Anemia becomes not the qualitative observation of pale skin, but the quantitative result of a laboratory test. When counting red cells was new, the act enumerating them was the responsibility of the patient's physician, sitting before a microscope, and soon thereafter of the physician's assistant or intern. Then came the clinical laboratory, where a technician, a stranger, tallies the cells; and then came a machine to do the counting. Now, the count is a number, an abstraction. The physician orders a test, and the next day brings a number. An abnormal number defines anemia.

The physician's gaze turns, generation by generation, from the patient, to the microscope, to the written page inscribed with numerals, to the computer monitor transiently inscribed with glowing phosphors.

This defines not one but two essential moments in medical history. The first is the point at which a qualitative clinical observation is replaced by a quantitative result from a machine, precise but abstract. The second is the point at which disease is defined not as an event of bad health, a badness in a person's physiology, a *hurt*, but a statistical *deviation from normalcy*. The modern physician has seen a thousand patients with anemia and a hundred with severe anemia, but rarely does the doctor describe them looking pale. In any event, studies have concluded that doctors are not all that skilled in detecting anemia from the observation of paleness, even when they *are* looking. Pallor has lost its valence as medical information. Never have I heard an intern say that the patient looks pale. Pale has no more meaning, now, than the four humors, or the aether, or phlogiston. Pale is not.

One more point: the modern physician will never know if a patient is anemic, unless by recourse to the machine, residing somewhere else, in a place apart.

6. What the Doctor Is Thinking

FOR AN AMERICAN PHYSICIAN OF THE TWENTY-FIRST century, anemia relates somehow to a lack of blood. The term, in our purportedly precise age, is surprisingly vague. It could mean too little blood in the entire body, as when one has hemorrhaged; or too few red blood cells in a given volume of blood; or too little of the hemoglobin molecule in a given volume of blood. Even the question of *too little* is not entirely clear—too little in comparison to what? To a numerical range, compared with other people? (Which other people? Defined by gender, age, nationality, race, ethnicity?) In comparison to a normal function? (Which function?)

A step more: compared *by whom*? By each individual physician? By some consensus of expert physicians? By a computer?

And yet one step more: conceived in terms of disease, or health?

Stop. The way a modern doctor *uses* the concept of anemia is this. He orders a blood test, checking a box on a paper form or on a computer pull-down menu. Then someone else, usually a technician hired specifically for this purpose, inserts a needle into the patient's arm and withdraws a sample of blood. A third person, a courier of some sort, transports the sample to a laboratory; a fourth person enters demographic and billing information; and a fifth person inserts the sample into a machine, which manipulates the specimen in various ways and produces several numbers. These feed into a computer, which reports the numbers to the physician.

This set of steps generates a set of numbers that the doctor interprets. These the doctor *must* interpret, for neglecting to interpret the data would be an unforgivable omission, a crime.

The numbers have names, which the doctor refers to basic concepts learned in medical school. Foremost among them is the hemoglobin concentration. Hemoglobin is the molecule that carries oxygen in the blood. It lives in a red blood cell, an erythrocyte, that flows in the bloodstream and whose entire function is to ferry hemoglobin. Red is the color of hemoglobin bound to oxygen. This compound, oxyhemoglobin, makes the red cell red, makes blood red, renders a ruddy complexion red, makes a maiden blush.

When anemia was a new idea, in the nineteenth century, the doctor would prick the patient's finger and examine the blood himself, using two techniques. One was to create a dried smear of blood on a glass slide, stain it chemically, and examine it under the microscope. The other was to place the blood, treated chemically so as to prevent clotting, in a minute chamber and count the cells, again under a microscope. The doctor performed these steps himself and therefore experienced the results directly, using his own hands and eyes, a corporeal knowing very different from the abstracting knowing of today. Then, one saw what one saw, albeit with special instruments; now, one sees numbers.

How does the doctor interpret the number? Most likely he will compare it to some normal range, seeing that a given result is below, within, or above the normal range. Whence these norms? They come from testing the blood of a thousand persons, or ten thousand, and deriving a statistical average defined in terms of standard deviations, a calculation that expresses the expected amount of variability in a group. In America, most laboratories calculate a normal range for hemoglobin concentration of about 14–18 g/dL in adult men, and 12–16 g/dL in adult women. (The units are grams per deciliter. A gram is about a thirtieth of an ounce, dry weight. A deciliter is about 3 liquid ounces.) Each laboratory, by the way, reports its own normal ranges, and each varies a little from the other, depending on its instruments and its population.

So that the doctor, seeing that our seventy-four-year-old man's hemoglobin measures 13 g/dL, concludes that the value is abnormal. Actually, the computerized printout helps the physician considerably in this regard by listing the abnormal values in a separate column. The busy clinician need only scan the page to see which results fall in the right-hand column, the abnormals, the worthy objects of his attention, topics of his scrutiny and further investigation. These abnormals command his entire regard, the normal results fall by the wayside as so much innocent and irrelevant chatter.

The physician phones or writes the patient, or an assistant or nurse phones or writes, or someone schedules a follow-up visit. We customarily learn lab results through calls or notes, but information that requires a follow-up visit conjures fear; the news must be serious indeed. Biopsy results, HIV results, genetic test results—these are the sort that can only be conveyed in person. You have cancer, you have AIDS, you have Huntington's disease—or you do not—these reports change your life, as is known to all the participants. Let us say here that the physician telephones. "Your blood results are back. You have mild anemia. There are many possible causes. I'd like to run some extra tests to see what the cause might be. Please stop by for these at your earliest convenience."

Doctors express their requests for further investigation in different ways. One physician might minimize his concern, *I'm sure it's nothing, but we have to check*, reducing his own anxiousness by shrinking the arena. *You're OK, I'm OK, lay your fears to rest.* Another takes the opposite approach, *There's something wrong with you and we have to find what it is*, finding an almost sadistic pleasure in condemning the patient to disease. *I am well and you are sick, hah!* The best might find a middle ground that expresses concern without inducing terror; but the patient, who functions simultaneously as interlocutor and as subject of the discussion, also modulates the terms of exchange, minimizing or maximizing according to his own fear and remonstrance.

Is the patient concerned? Undoubtedly yes. For the patient well knows that the ordinary consequence of a lab test is a report that *everything is fine*. Years of the annual physical exam, in pediatric and adult life, have taught him that. A test that must be repeated or investigated further must mean that something is wrong, and perhaps something is terribly wrong. *Doctor, what is wrong?*

The doctor responds that he doesn't know yet, and indeed he doesn't. More tests are required.

Which tests? Again, the doctor might take a minimalist or a maximalist approach. The former would be simply to repeat the test. This is convenient and cheap if the repeat value is normal, but inconvenient and dissatisfying if not. ("Cheap" also begs the questions of whose cost, expressed how, paid by whom. The cost of a test might be borne by the patient, the insurer, the hospital, or the government. Its cost, its price, and its charge may all be different. Meanwhile, a return visit costs the patient time, money, and maybe lost wages.) The latter, maximalist approach would be to test for many causes of anemia off the bat. This seems brilliant if it identifies an unusual condition rapidly, but silly and maybe irresponsible if everything turns out normal, or if a simple cause is found at great expense.

The psychiatrists speak of underpathologizing and over-pathologizing. To underpathologize is to deem important symptoms to be probably innocuous, while to overpathologize is to assign disease categories to life's simpler ups and downs. Is a teen's sadness ordinary turmoil or major depression? A diagnostician might habitually lean to one side or the other of such difficult distinctions, and thus be called an under- or overpathologizer.

Medical thinking draws the doctor to the abnormal. Normal is unworthy of notice, boring, pleasant but inconsequential. Abnormal is noteworthy, interesting, unpleasant but consequential.

A medical fact is called a *finding*. A finding is something discovered about a patient that warrants thought or action, and this something is almost always aberrant, a deviation from the expected, an abnormal. An enlarged liver is a finding, a normal-sized liver is not.

It is Augustine, I think, who somewhere writes that literature deals with vice because virtue is always the same, unitary and boring, while vice is multitudinous, multifarious, multidimensional, fascinating. It was certainly he who worried out loud that he concerned himself more for Dido, a fiction, than for his own soul.

Medicine thus draws the physician away from health and toward disease.

To the doctor, anemia means a deviation from normal that demands explanation. Implicit in this construct are four concepts.

1. What is normal? Normal can be considered in terms of what *is*, a statistical concept of averages and variation, or in terms of what *should be*, a valuative concept of ethics and morals. The former concerns knowledge, the latter judgment.

If we measured the height of all the men in New York City, we would generate a list of perhaps four million numbers. We could average these numbers and state the average height of New York men. We could manipulate the figures further to derive additional conclusions: the median height of the group, the standard deviation of their height (how much the measurements tended to vary). We could use the latter to derive a normal range, such that ninety-five percent of the men were within that range. They are said to be normal. Anyone above or below the range is said to be abnormal.

The process, though it seems so simple, is fraught with difficulty. We cannot measure all the men, so instead we measure some of the men and extrapolate regarding the entire group. Did we miss some kinds of men more than others? (For example, homeless men, or immigrants suspicious of official-looking measurers.) Should we include or exclude the old men, who are not so tall as once they were? The stooped men, the sick men, the men in hospitals?

Beyond the statistical calculation of averages and ranges, there is a valuative component that assigns relative worth to various measurements. A man whose height is below the normal range is short. Short is bad. How short is bad, and how bad is short? Is short a disease? Presidents are not often short. Should I give my son medicine to make him taller, so that he can be president?

Tall, viewed statistically, is just as abnormal as short. But viewed as a value, tall is good. Well, but not too tall. Too tall is great for basketball, sometimes, but problematic otherwise: awkward in theaters and inconvenient in clothing stores; also mismatched in ardor and painfully predisposed to arthritis and backache. Too tall may be a giant, a freak.

Anemia could be defined in the same way, and usually is. The clinical pathologists take a group of healthy persons, perform the blood test, and derive a series of numbers, from which calculations are derived concerning means, medians, standard deviations, ranges, and so on. These can be subdivided according to gender, age, race, ethnicity, etc. In this schema, anyone falling outside the normal range of hemoglobin measurements is said to be abnormal. A man whose hemoglobin measurement is below the normal range has anemia. Anemia is bad. How anemic is bad? When is anemia a disease, and when an inconsequential variation from the expected norm?

The elderly often have hemoglobin values below the "normal" range, even when they appear healthy otherwise. Does this mean that they are sick, suffering from some as-yet undetected disease, or might the declining hemoglobin number be a "normal" consequence of normal aging, comparable to balding?

The discussion of normal and abnormal can easily become circular. Thus Galen, the renowned physician of the Roman era whose treatises dominated European and Muslim medicine for a millennium: "In healthy people all indications are normal; in people suffering disease, they are abnormal, to the extent to which the person is diseased."

2. What is deviation? Social critics and philosophers have shown how science and medicine, in defining such concepts as normalcy and health, can be enlisted as agents of social dominance and control. Indeed, although a statistic appears objective and value-neutral, the word initially denoted information in the service of the state, especially in the areas of civic administration and finance. The first statistics were political arithmetic, and so they were called.

About twenty percent of the population is left-handed. Left-handedness is now considered, in principle, a normal variation without any positive or negative value assigned. True, a left-handed person might suffer little inconveniences when confronting the right-handed world of borrowed baseball gloves, high school armrests, hand tools, guitars, and so on. Still, the situation feels very different from the one obtaining two generations ago, when a left-handed child was forced to write and throw with the right hand. As it turned out, a child so forced often developed a stutter. Trying to convert the child from left-handed to right-handed, from bad to good, the parents and teachers committed violence against him that resulted in something unequivocally bad, the stammer. Even now, the old valuations survive by clinging to old words and phrases: *sinister*, bad; *dexterous*, good; *a left-handed compliment*, bad. One shakes with the right hand, salutes with the right, eats (in many countries of Africa and Asia) only with the right.

Anemia, though defined as a statistical deviation from a numerical norm, seems as though it should be bad. Bad because deviant? Bad because falling short of some ideal? Bad because unhealthy? Bad because tinged with a suspect air of wrongdoing, or evil?

3. Deviance demands explanation. The doctor may or may not be concerned about the abnormal test result. Often, such a result is essentially meaningless, an oddity of the day or of the lab, a transient aberration that the body will correct on its own, a passing infection, a fleeting environmental insult. Nonetheless, the doctor feels bound to pursue an explanation. Bound how or by whom, one might ask. First is a set of clinical customs that place a premium on determining a diagnosis. (His own curiosity or indifference may play a role.) Second is a legal system that would find him at fault if ever a condition were to arise that was not adequately investigated. (His own sense of vulnerability or invulnerability may play a role.) Both imperatives are open to question. Different clinical customs might instead prioritize treatment, for example, or comfort. A different legal system might instead recognize intention, or acknowledge that some imperfections may yet be blameless.

4. *What is medical number?* The Pythagoreans of the fifth century BCE loved number, above all its purity, an absolute truth that stood above mundane contingencies. Scientists, drawn to measurement since the Renaissance, have loved numbers differently. Medicine takes part in this latter fascination and measures the body and its functions. Modern medical knowing has become a process of quantification. Health and illness have come to consist in numbers: blood pressure, blood count, serum cholesterol, a thousand such. The patient is not fat, his body-mass index is elevated above some cutoff. A treatment works depending on how the numbers work out: a score increases or decreases, a proportion is greater or lesser.

William Thomson, Lord Kelvin, for whom the temperature scale was named, writes that "when you can measure what you are speaking about and express it in numbers you know something about it; but when you cannot measure it, when you cannot express it in numbers, your knowledge is of a meager and unsatisfactory kind: it may be the beginning of knowledge, but you have scarcely, in your thoughts, advanced to the state of *science*, whatever the matter may be." And yet the position does not always hold in clinical medicine. Consider Paul Ehrlich, one of the great early hematologists, writing a few years later: "As matters stand at present the clinician must be warned against the introduction into practice of uncertain methods of examination which yield varying results. The very fact that the results are expressed in figures awakens a false appearance of accuracy, which should be avoided even more than the utilization of subjective methods of examination."

Medicine can never aspire to the purity of Pythagorean number, but so too must it proceed cautiously in assigning too many of the body's secrets to quantification. The instruments, after all, are only so accurate, can only perform as we have instructed them, and can only measure what we have learned to measure.

Anemia joins all these senses of medical wrongness, defining a place where disparate notions of abnormality come together. Anemia is a numerical aberrancy, a departure from normal, a departure from ordinary, a departure from sameness, a defiance, an unwellness, maybe a momentary fluke, maybe a catastrophe. But the doctor, confronting an abnormal number, feels bound to investigate. Thus he embarks, and causes the patient to embark, on the diagnostic journey.

7. Diagnostic Ceremonies

ANEMIA: ITS SIGNIFICANCE COULD RANGE FROM INNOCENT to fatal, from nothing to everything. In a young woman, anemia stems most likely from iron deficiency, the result of menstrual blood loss coupled with inadequate dietary iron. In an older person, anemia raises the specter of cancer or leukemia.

The doctor who discovers anemia must notify the patient and arrange for further testing. To consider the options for notifying the patient one by one:

1. The doctor phones the patient. This has several advantages. Dialogue allows both doctor and patient to ask questions and to voice their concerns. However, phoning takes a lot of time. Often there is a chain of message leaving with answering machines, voice-mail, workplace assistants, or family members. Each of these breaches confidentiality in greater or lesser measure, since even the fact of a doctor's message is a little out of the ordinary and might mean *something*. In addition, the patient has no record of what the doctor actually said and often misremembers or misconstrues the discussion. The doctor, of course, must keep a record of the call, often typing or scribbling away rather than focusing on the discussion at hand.

2. The doctor writes the patient. This loses the advantages of dialogue but creates a record for both parties and gen-

erally takes less time than the telephone for a physician skilled in typing or dictation.

3. A nurse or assistant telephones the patient. This allows for limited dialogue, depending on circumstance. It works best (a) when the results are normal, or (b) when the caller is particularly trained in the topic under discussion.

4. The doctor e-mails the patient. E-mail generates a particular genre of writing, just as the telegram once did. Its style is more casual than the formal letter, resembling an informal note more than a missive. E-mail also tends toward a rapid, back-and-forth banter, a form of electronic tennis played with a low net. Confidentiality issues again arise.

5. A follow-up visit is scheduled to discuss test results. This takes the event to a whole new level, raising the stakes. *It must be serious*, or *it could be serious*, or *there's something too big for the telephone*.

If the patient is a woman below the age of about fifty, give or take, the physician thinks first of iron deficiency. A menstruating woman bleeds. The blood consists of cells and proteins and fluid, and the cells consist primarily of iron. To bleed is to lose iron. Unless she ingests iron in fairly substantial amounts, whether in food or tablet form, a menstruating woman develops iron deficiency and becomes anemic.

The diagnostic ceremony surrounding iron-deficiency anemia broaches two subjects that fall outside customary patient-physician discourse. The first concerns the menses. Doctors are trained to ask a woman about her periods, but generally they do so cautiously, if at all. "And your periods— fairly regular?" he might ask, midway between one thing and another, an informal question, a "by the way," rather than a primary interrogative. The doctor's focus is regularity, for irregularity might indicate hormonal disregulation, disease, or incipient menopause. The woman might also talk about flow—heavy, light, in between—but how defined?

How many tampons or pads a day? Where do the patient and the physician develop their notions of normal, and whether the patient bleeds more or less than the putative norm? One would rather not talk about it. Even the medical professor, meeting with students, jokes the question aside, or else opines in high-serious posture.

The second concerns diet. Again, doctors are supposed to ask their patients about their nutrition, but this is a tedious and troubled undertaking. *What do you eat?* Are we talking about today, or this week, or generally? How does one respond? What one likes to eat? What one eats habitually? How does one specify amounts? No one answers very truthfully. It feels like a test, and one exaggerates the "good foods" (meaning, these days, protein, vegetables, fruits, and whole grains) and underplays the "bad foods" (fats, sugars, and refined carbohydrates). Inquiring about iron intake, the physician might ask about dietary intake of meats, but "red meat" has been villainized by the cholesterol movement. The patient who wants to please the doctor and to please herself mentally reduces her red-meat intake. Other foods contain relatively little iron. Beans, yes, but how many of us eat lentils and kidney beans on a regular basis? Dark leafy vegetables, yes, but how many of us eat these more than once or twice a month? Give us this day our daily kale? Our broccoli rabe? Spinach is healthy—or was, until the *E. coli* scare of 2006— but spinach as a source of iron is mainly fiction.

How much iron must a woman take in? This is a hard number to come by. The Food and Nutrition Board of the Institute of Medicine has determined that adult women before menopause should take in about eighteen milligrams of iron per day, contrasted with eight milligrams per day for men. Those are fine numbers that translate readily into prescriptions or pills, but how do they translate into dietary recommendations? The textbooks of medicine skirt the issue by speaking of "the average Western diet" and "a balanced diet" without specifying what these are. Eight ounces of meat a day? Half that? Twice that? In fact, there is a considerable range of meat intake between the urban vegetarian and the rural carnivore, and between those who have heeded the government-sponsored recommendation to reduce intake of "red meat" and those who haven't.

A little homework calculates that eighteen mg of iron would require about a pound of steak. Well, there are alternative sources. The same eighteen milligrams of iron could be found in nineteen ounces of roast turkey, four pounds of canned tuna, two-plus cups of boiled lentils, three cups of cooked spinach, or twenty slices of enriched bread. A pregnant woman, by the way, needs about half again as much iron: one and a half pounds of steak daily, three cups of lentils, and so on. A vegetarian also needs twice the usual amount, for the iron derived from plants is not so well absorbed.

One pictures the juicy steak, the rare roast beef *saignant*, rosy, and thinks that their virtue must lie in eating or drinking blood itself. Football players eat steak on the eve of the big game, as soldiers once did before battle. Victorious warriors once drank the blood of vanquished foes, and successful hunters drank the blood of their freshly slain prey. But the iron in meat consists not so much in blood as in myoglobin, the main meat protein, rich in iron. The iron in myoglobin gives meat its characteristic red color—and indeed, it is usually iron that gives the red color to nearly everything you can think of, from red rocks to red planets to red apples to red meat. Iron from myoglobin is not only the most abundant (potential) dietary source of the mineral but also the easiest for the body to absorb; one digests flesh better than rocks, and iron tablets contain the rock form.

In the strange behavior called pica, people (usually women) eat substances generally considered inedible, typically small

granular material such as dirt, clay, starch, and laundry deter-
gent. The name comes from the Latin for magpie, that thiev-
ing black bird who is supposed to eat anything. The practice is
an old one that can be documented from Hippocratic times,
fifth century BCE, until the present. (In one of the stories
embedded in *Don Quixote*, the narrator speaks of having such
an illness, so disturbed that he eats "earth, plaster, coal and
other worse things.") The modern interpretation of pica is
that persons so afflicted have iron-deficiency anemia, which
compels them to seek out iron even in its most rudimentary
forms, such as soil. One might well question whether this con-
fident biochemical explanation entirely comprehends this
eccentric compulsive eating behavior, which, from a different
vantage, resembles anorexia nervosa or bulimia.

When we were in medical school, the professors taught
that pica was mainly a problem of poor, malnourished black
women in the South. Their claims may stand scrutiny. Ethnol-
ogists have found that eating clay is a culturally accepted
practice in certain parts of Africa, especially during pregnancy.
Moreover, eating clay may have particular pharmacologic
benefits. Strange diseases, and especially strange behaviors,
happen mainly to persons unlike ourselves.

And how might the physician ask his anemic patient
whether she is eating dirt? How might she tell him, were she
so inclined?

Facing a young woman with anemia, should the physician test at all? Perhaps it is more sensible to treat with iron
and see what happens. An improved blood count after a few
months of iron therapy would confirm the diagnosis. But
there are problems with this common approach. First, some
women will have a different cause of anemia, such as sickle-
cell trait or thalassemia trait, and they should know about
these genetic conditions before they bear children. Second,

iron supplements are difficult to take. They cause constipation and other forms of gastrointestinal upset. And so, the doctor requests an additional test. *Please come back to the office at your convenience, you have anemia, I would like to check your iron level.* The test is performed, the result confirms the initial impression, the tablets are prescribed. It has been a simple, straightforward, and entirely satisfactory transaction. The stakes, after all, were pretty low.

If the patient is not a menstruating woman, iron deficiency means something entirely different. This person must also be bleeding, but where? Unless there is some clearly identifiable source, such as a recent surgical operation or blood donation, the occult bleeding usually has arisen from the gastrointestinal tract, which must therefore be interrogated. ("What!" says the patient, "but I'm not bleeding!" "Ah," responds the physician, "the blood loss can be tiny and invisible, I intuit what none can see.") The doctor refers such a patient to the gastroenterologist, who will perform colonoscopy and upper endoscopy. These procedures, now well known, involve the insertion of long, flexible, fiber-optic instruments into the rectum and mouth, respectively, to see the insides of the intestines and stomach directly. If these tests are unrevealing, the next step is direct examination of the small intestine, either by a special endoscopic examination or by means of a minute camera that the patient swallows (capsule enteroscopy).

Here, the stakes are much higher. What the doctor is looking for, whether he says so or not, is cancer. True, there are other causes of occult gastrointestinal bleeding, benign polyps and vascular malformations in the intestine, ulcers and gastritis in the stomach, but colon cancer is the main focus of attention. The savvy patient infers this message, sensing that the doctor seems rather more urgent about the colonoscopy than he had about previous tests.

So grave are the implications of iron deficiency in this setting that they enter the legal domain. The doctor who fails to recommend colonoscopy for the patient (male or postmenopausal female) with iron deficiency may have committed malpractice.

And if the anemic patient does not have iron deficiency, what then? Now the doctor must begin to pry. Sickle-cell anemia, common in persons of African descent and in certain others, is a genetic disorder of the hemoglobin molecule. A person with two affected genes will suffer recurrent episodes of severe pain. A person with only one affected gene has sickle trait, a benign condition that causes mild anemia or nothing at all. Somewhat similar is thalassemia, a different hemoglobin mutation that affects people from lands adjoining the Mediterranean (hence the name, from the Greek *thalassa*, sea) as well as India and East Asia. Again, persons with only one affected gene have thalassemia trait, resulting in mild anemia.

Vitamin B12, cyanocobalamin, is an indispensable but ubiquitous substance that is found abundantly in all animal products, including flesh of any source, milk, and eggs. However, people as they age often lose the ability to absorb this vitamin efficiently. About twenty percent of the population develops this condition after the age of sixty-five. The consequence of B12 deficiency is a certain form of anemia as well as problems in digestive and nervous systems, including decreased sensation, "pins and needles," visual loss, personality changes, and dementia. Before the disease was understood and treatment became available, its natural history was an inexorable march to death— hence its somber name, pernicious anemia. A series of Nobel Prizes went to the physician-scientists who figured it all out.

And if not these, what? Most likely the bone marrow is not performing its proper job in manufacturing blood cells. In the so-called anemia of chronic disease, some illness not directly related to blood formation is suppressing this function. Examples might include rheumatoid arthritis or tuberculosis. Otherwise, the problem is a condition of the bone marrow itself. Usually this means some acquired mutation of a precursor cell, one whose offspring are the red and white blood cells. These conditions, the refractory anemias or myelodysplastic syndromes, may ultimately change to a form of leukemia. If so, they resist treatment and typically prove fatal. Sometimes, of course, the discovery of anemia leads to an immediate diagnosis of leukemia or another hematologic malignancy, such as multiple myeloma.

Evaluation of the bone marrow requires a different subspecialist, a hematologist, who will perform a bone marrow biopsy. This test involves the insertion of a small needle—but not small enough, the patient might say—into the bone of the pelvis. The patient lies prone, the hematologist numbs the skin and drills his hollow probe into the bone. It hurts, but not so very much more than dental work. The test, nonetheless, is regarded as fearful, like the lumbar puncture (spinal tap). Why? Perhaps there is something particular about needles placed in the back, where the patient can't see—*what is he really doing to me?*

And if all these tests are normal? The sagacious doctor resolves to wait and see.

Is anemia ever normal? Certainly, the person with mild anemia will feel no ill consequence of the reduced blood count. If the anemia signals a disease, best to know about it. And if an exhaustive search discovers no disease?

Doctors sometimes invoke a secret reassurance called "normal for you." Implied in the concept is a finding or test result that is outside the normal range for people in general, but satisfactory for the patient at hand. It seems not to connote disease, or if it does then the disease is not apparent, or not yet apparent, or not (yet) requiring action, or not important enough to warrant further testing. This breast lump might be worrisome in someone else, but you have always had it, it is normal for you. Your hemoglobin measurement is low but has always been so, the tests are all normal, it is normal for you. Abnormal in medicine is usually bad but can be mollified if it is of long standing. A recent change from normal to abnormal cannot be mollified. Medicine views change with suspicion, it ranks among the conservative professions.

The average blood count of older persons is lower than that of their younger successors. This demographic observation could be interpreted in two ways. Either the elderly are becoming sick, as indeed they may be, or a decline in hemoglobin is a normal concomitant of aging. Medicine, officially, rejects the latter position. And yet the practicing physician often looks the other way when discovering mild anemia in a patient past middle age. If the preliminary tests are normal, especially iron and B12 but often the test for myeloma as well, one resolves to monitor the blood test periodically without more aggressive investigation. It would serve little purpose to diagnose myelodysplastic syndrome, for which no definitive treatment is available, only to tell the patient that she has an incurable blood disease that is likely to turn to leukemia, if only she lives long enough. Indeed, she is likely to die of something else first, rendering the dire hematologic diagnosis irrelevant.

General physicians perform most of these tests in their own offices, or in nearby commercial laboratories. ("Commercial laboratories," we say, as if the doctor's office were not a place of commerce. Perhaps the difference is that the companies that perform blood tests do so explicitly as a business, and the doctor only implicitly.) A well-informed generalist will consult a subspecialist to perform special "invasive" tests, such as colonoscopy and bone marrow biopsy, or occasionally when otherwise stumped. The generalist who discovers anemia and refers the patient immediately to a hematologist, as if by reflex, isn't doing much thinking and certainly isn't providing the patient with a comprehensive model of care. And yet how often one sees this mentality of *problem equals consultation*: chest pain, see a cardiologist; cough, see a pulmonologist; sneeze, see an allergist, and so on.

Medical custom and regulation place no restriction on the tests that a doctor can order—with a few exceptions. An insurance company might refuse to pay for a test, but this does not prevent the patient from undergoing the test and paying for it personally. The two exceptions to the unrestricted nature of medical tests involve those for HIV/AIDS and for genetic disorders.

To test a patient for hepatitis, for example, the doctor checks a box on a computer screen or a laboratory requisition slip. A technician draws the blood, the sample goes to a lab, the lab reports the result to the physician, the physician informs the patient. (Odd: the lab does not report results directly to patients, who are not the purported clients, even though they pay the fees, directly or indirectly. Perhaps the workflow model imagines that the patients couldn't handle the news without the intermediary physicians.)

Other tests involve a small ceremony: fasting. Before testing for diabetes or cholesterol disorders, the physician may ask the patient to skip all food for perhaps twelve hours. In practice, this means fasting overnight. For most persons of modern secular society, this is the *only* occasion for fasting. But the overnight fast is an ancient ritual of consecration and dedication, the knight-errant before his ordeal, the shaman before his vision quest, the penitent, the novitiate, the holy man, the sage.

Testing for HIV is different, strictly regulated by the states. In New York, for example, the physician must counsel the patient before performing the test and after the results have come back. The instructions recommend twenty minutes for each session. The doctor informs the patient of the basics of the HIV virus and its transmission, the utility of the test, the possibility of erroneous results or erroneous conclusions, and the importance of barrier contraception. Furthermore, they must discuss the benefits of HIV testing, including the advantages of early detection and treatment, as well as the risks of testing, including the possibility of stigmatization, prejudice, and discrimination. Finally, after discussing the confidentiality of the test, the doctor must inform the patient that he must report a positive test to the State Department of Health, which in turn will write the patient regarding possible "contacts" who may also be infected.

The physician must give the patient a four-page information brochure, downloadable from the Internet, and then ask the patient to sign a paper of "informed consent." The laboratory may require the patient to sign an additional form before accepting the blood for analysis.

At the second visit, when the patient returns to learn the results, the physician must again provide about twenty minutes of counseling regarding the significance of the result, the treatment options if positive, the need for continued preventive measures if negative.

This diagnostic ritual began, as so often they do, with a rational foundation. When testing for HIV first became available, a positive result was a virtual death sentence. No cure was available (and still isn't), and no treatment was effective (but now is). Members of gay advocacy groups argued, with justification, that to be known as HIV positive, or even as someone who had undergone HIV testing, could bring significant adverse repercussions. Would such persons be publicly identified? Would they be quarantined, rounded up? Would they be able to obtain health insurance, life insurance, disability insurance? Would they lose their jobs, would their homes be picketed, would they be hounded out of town? The groups pushed to safeguard anonymity. In those early days, a numbered sticker went on the tube of blood, an identical sticker on the patient's chart, and no one knew the match but the ordering physician. The Department of Health, meanwhile, introduced the other provisions, the admonitions about transmission, the partner notification, and so on.

And yet—twenty minutes, twice, forty minutes. The doctor's office usually allots some twenty or thirty minutes to the complete annual physical exam, sometimes more when the patient is paying more, sometimes less when the office is a for-profit concern or a clinic for the poor. Is HIV testing as important, nay twice as important, as the entire remainder of the health evaluation? If the result is positive, perhaps yes. But the result is almost always negative (i.e., normal, no infection).

The HIV test has been ritualized. A doctor might tell a patient that she has metastatic lung cancer, that she has but a few months to live, with less ceremony than discussing a normal result in an eminently treatable condition. The fanfare sets the HIV test, and hence HIV infection itself, apart from anything else in medicine. Granted, when HIV was new, it did seem apart from everything else, although now it is a chronic infection among others, not conceptually different from hepatitis C, for example, and not too different from such chronic noninfectious diseases as diabetes mellitus. Granted, too, the magnified nature of HIV testing tends to raise awareness of this major health problem. But the downside of the ritual is to create a barrier to HIV testing. Doctors perform the test too infrequently. About half the people in the United States with HIV infection don't know it, and presumably these are the ones most likely to spread the virus to others. Thus, ritualizing the HIV test tends to backfire against the very impulse that created the ritual, causing more people to go untested, more people to harbor undiagnosed infection, more opportunity to infect others, and wider spread of the epidemic.

Hepatitis C—a newly discovered disease proves in time to be treatable and manageable. HIV—a newly discovered disease proves in time to be treatable and manageable. Both involve infections with slowly moving viruses, both are transmitted mainly by sex and by intravenous drug use using contaminated paraphernalia. But what a difference in their social meaning and in their testing. Hepatitis was first known as something that happens, a disease among others, one that results perhaps from unsociable (or too sociable) behaviors, but not particularly valenced. HIV was first known as gay plague, a scourge. To test for hepatitis is to check a box. To test for HIV is to engage in a publicly mandated, privately performed ceremony.

The state also regulates testing for genetic conditions. These belong to three main types.

Testing for a condition called hemochromatosis exemplifies the first type. This is the commonest hereditary disorder of Caucasians, affecting about five per thousand. (The prevalence in other groups has been little studied—interestingly enough.) It causes its bearers to absorb iron excessively, which causes damage to the liver, heart, and other organs. Thus, when evaluating a patient with liver problems, the physician frequently tests for hemochromatosis. To do so, he must lead the patient through a process of informed consent, a highly abbreviated form of the process for HIV testing. In practice, the doctor fills out an extra form and checks a box, the patient signs, and the rest resembles any ordinary test.

The second type involves prenatal testing for hereditary disorders. This pertains mostly to Jews of eastern European extraction, the Ashkenazi. They, more than others, bear increased susceptibility to several important genetic diseases, including Tay-Sachs disease, Canavan's disease, and a number of others. A newly married couple or an expectant parent of such ancestry will frequently undergo genetic screening for these conditions. Again, doctor and patient must sign certain forms, but the test feels otherwise fairly routine. Commercial laboratories simplify the process by offering the tests together in a single package. The association with the sacraments of marriage and childbirth adds an extra emotive force. So too do some of the usually unspoken ramifications of a positive test result: the possibility of bearing a malformed child, or even one doomed to debility and premature death; the decision whether to terminate the pregnancy.

The third type of genetic testing is unique in all of medicine. Most cases of breast cancer occur more or less at random. That is, most women with breast cancer have no specific genetic susceptibility to this disease, as far as can be known. However, some women belong to families in which many members develop breast cancer. In recent years, two genes have been identified that, when present in abnormal (mutated) form, dramatically increase the likelihood of developing breast cancer. These genes, called BRCA–1 and –2, ordinarily code for proteins that correct errors in cell replication. If a woman inherits a mutated form of BRCA–1 or –2, her risk of developing breast cancer by age seventy is estimated at perhaps seventy-five percent, and ovarian cancer at about sixty percent.

Testing for BRCA mutations is now available. But a doctor can't order these tests from the office. Instead, the doctor refers the patient to a genetic counselor. The first meeting takes about an hour. The counselor outlines the patient's family history, explains basic genetics, discusses the BRCA genes, and provides an overview of decisions to be made should the test result be unfavorable. The counselor and the patient sign papers. The patient pays cash, up-front, twice: a check to the laboratory, a check to the counselor's office, for insurance companies typically accept no responsibility for such testing. Only one lab in the United States performs the test; it holds the patent. Then, the patient waits—although an extra fee of a few hundred dollars will provide rush service.

The patient waits. It takes about a month to reach the second meeting with the counselor, now accompanied by a physician. The patient strains to read the geneticists' expressions—the hint of a smile, a suppressed frown, what are they about to tell me? The door closes, all sit down, the counselor opens the folder and delivers the result.

The news may be big. A woman with positive results is well advised to have her ovaries surgically removed, before they can become cancerous. She will have extra-intensive screening for breast cancer, including such tests as annual MRIs, although insurance companies again may decline to pay for these. Her sisters and her cousins should undergo BRCA testing. And her daughters—what shall she tell them, and at what age?

Odd, though, that only the genetic counselor can perform the test. A general physician can order any other test available, including ones with far more import than BRCA testing. An abnormal result, remember, means only a *susceptibility* to certain cancers. The general physician must often tell patients that they *have* cancer, not just a susceptibility to cancer, and must also tell them that the disease is not curable, that they will die. Why should this information be treated as medical routine, and BRCA testing as so exceptional that none but the specially trained may order it?

First, a woman likely has feelings about breast cancer that are very different from anything she thinks or feels about iron overload or Canavan's disease. The breasts are objects of lavish or fetish attention, quite unlike any other body part. To lose an arm or an eye is a calamity, to lose a testicle a hardship but anyway men have two, to lose a kidney a mechanical surgical procedure, invisible once complete. But to lose a breast is a disfigurement, a slash, a sacrifice of the most visible external expression of adult femininity and sexuality.

Such feelings intensify and morph for the woman whose several relatives have had breast cancer, the woman with "a positive family history of breast cancer." She has seen her mother, grandmother, aunts, and great aunts suffer and die, or she has heard their stories, or their legends—for young women dying become in families the stuff of legend, saints, martyrs, guardian angels. They pray for you, they watch over you, they will welcome you with open arms in the oneday bosom of Abraham. Breast cancer for such a woman may seem an inevitability, a destiny, to join her late progenitors in the fatal march toward doom. To test for BRCA is to bring these issues, a lifetime of issues, a deathtime of issues, all to bear at once.

Genetics and predestination? The Horatio Alger American believes that we all determine our own destinies, that hard work and pluck will overcome any hardship, that we all are self-made men, or so we can become. The Puritan American recalls his Calvinist heritage: our actions have no bearing whatsoever on our eventual salvation or damnation, all is foreordained and quite outside our influence. Genetics sounds more like John Calvin than Ragged Dick and Tattered Tom. To inherit the gene, one thinks, is to inherit the fate. No, says the kind genetic counselor, that is not what I meant at all, that is not it at all. But what kind words could overthrow a lifetime of ingrained ecclesiastical ordinances?

III. ANEMIC KNOWING

Every era and every place construct an understanding of the body and its mechanisms. The body's parts and functions are laced within a system known differently in time and place: the five elements of Chinese medicine, the four humors of Greco-Roman medicine, the three humors of Ayurvedic medicine, the dualistic oppositions of modern biomedicine, the unity of so-called holistic medicine and its many avatars. Within such systems, certain organs assume a privileged status, thus the heart, the liver, the eyes and ears, the genitalia. Within the system of the blood, the spleen and the marrow both stand apart, mythic and supreme.

8. Spleen

Spleen, splenetic, splenic, splenic anemia, splenic.
Spleen, an organ, spleen, an animosity.
Spleen, a disposition, fretful, peevish, melancholic, heartful,
    black bile.
Spleen, splanchnic, innards, guts.

THE SPLEEN IS AN ORGAN. IT RESIDES IN THE LEFT UPPER quadrant of the abdomen, just beneath the ribs. It lives there silently. All of us are aware of our hearts, our lungs, our intestines, our genitalia, our eyes and ears and nose and mouth, but none perceives his spleen. It dwells submerged, beneath the threshold of consciousness. It serves a vegetative function, in the old parlance.

Textbooks of anatomy depict the spleen as a shapeless lump of flesh, unworthy of detailed regard. Early encyclopedias enroll the spleen among the "ductless glands," together with the thyroid, the parathyroids, and the adrenals. A gland's function is to secrete, a secretion must pass down a duct, who could imagine a ductless gland, a function without a function? Kant, echoing Aristotle, said that everything must have a function, nothing exists otherwise, to discover a new organ in the body would invoke a search for its function, how might a gland with no port serve?

The spleen warrants attention only insofar as it malfunctions. The spleen is enlarged: anemia. Rarely is the spleen enlarged for long without anemia, and what might be the connection?

Ancient of days, the man looked pale, the spleen was enlarged, why. We moderns might say that disease was malaria, the spleen is enlarged, plasmodium parasites have invaded the body, they break apart the red blood cells, anemia ensues, the spleen enlarged to process the busted cells.

Modern times, new mechanisms, the spleen is enlarged, the patient is anemic, malaria, maybe, what else comes to mind, lymphoma, leukemia, thalassemia, chronic hemolytic anemia, nasty diseases, technical diseases, who shall understand them.

Take out the spleen, surgery, major surgery, who shall decide.

The spleen is an organ. It resides in the left upper quadrant of the abdomen. We name its function, a materialist view, not precisely its purpose, a teleological view. Its function, as best we moderns understand it, is twofold. (1) It serves as a giant lymph node, the greatest of the body, it helps to fight infection. Just as a lymph node in the neck might enlarge in response to strep throat, a regional defense against a local infection, so might the spleen enlarge in response to infectious mononucleosis, a systemic defense against a global infection. (2) It processes old red blood cells. A red cell lives for ninety days, give or take, and when it is old and gray and full of sleep the spleen recognizes its senectitude and takes it aside, takes it down, administers some fatal blow and breaks it apart, recycles its parts for future use, its iron and vital stuff. Thus speaks each of us; and when the cells are short-lived, for whatever reason or whatever disease, the recycling must quicken apace, and the spleen must enlarge to perform its accelerated duties.

The two functions compete against each other. A spleen that enlarges to fight infection may capture healthy red cells and induce anemia. A spleen that enlarges to process dying red cells may fight infection inadequately. Details, details, medicine is never far from its details, the spleen is especially important in fighting certain infections, we think, the man with a malfunctioning or absent spleen should receive vaccine against pneumonia, should avoid the haunts of Babesia, an infection common in the offshore islands of New England but not elsewhere, Nantucket, Martha's Vineyard, Shelter Island, go not there if your spleen is awry.

The spleen enlarges in lymphoma and leukemia, the hematologic system has run amok, the white cells proliferate unseemingly, the red cells are suppressed, anemia. An adult with an enlarged spleen is always sick, often severely sick, often mortally sick.

The doctor always examines the spleen, or seeks it out. Whether you are well or ill, the examiner lays hands in the left upper quadrant of the abdomen, take a deep breath. One can usually feel the spleen in normal children; in healthy adults, rarely or never. Palpable spleen (adult) = disease. Take a deep breath.

The doctor who can feel the spleen of a seemingly healthy adult knows instantly that something serious is amiss. This man is sick, though he feel well, though he feel a thousand times well. Something is seriously wrong. Secret and unwelcome knowledge, as indeed the physician's knowledge is so often secret and unwelcome, fatal blemish, fatal augury cast for those I have loved.

Palpable spleen and ancient disease, malaria, hepatitis. Palpable spleen and Victorian disease, tuberculosis, Keats, Chopin, Violetta, Mimi. Palpable spleen and modern disease, AIDS, cancer, scourge.

Spleen, sorcery. Among the Gusii people of southwest Kenya, an autopsy is performed whenever witchcraft is suspected as a cause of death. Finding that the spleen is enlarged —as often happens in malarial regions, witchcraft or no— confirms the diagnosis.

*   *   *

First comes spleen, an organ in the left upper quadrant of the abdomen. From that word derives "*splanchnon*," innards, guts, the inner organs. Carnivorous man prefers skeletal muscle, loin, filet, ham, haunch. Viewed gastronomically, the splanchna are the less desirable parts, fit for sausage and maybe stews, stuffing, giblets; or, paradoxically, as delicacies for the discerning or the adventurous or the sated, sweetbreads; or something that partakes of both, Mr Leopold Bloom ate with relish the inner organs of beasts and fowls.

The earliest thinkers of the Greek world, called presocratics by postsocratics, discovered an idea—or they invented or posited it—the idea of polar binary opposites, hot ↔ cold, wet ↔ dry. Later thinkers, above all, Aristotle, codified this into a fourfold template, like a cross inscribed in a circle, like the four points of a compass. Thinking of the universe, these corresponded to the symmetry of the four elements, fire, air, earth, water. Thinking of the body, the intersections of these four attributes became four humors, which in turn could correspond to four body fluids. Thus:

$$hot + dry = phlegm$$
$$hot + wet = blood$$
$$cold + dry = bile$$
$$cold + wet = \ldots what?$$

Search and search in vain, there is no fourth fluid to complete the pattern. I have seen blood, I have seen phlegm, the discharge of the nose, maybe of the brain. I have seen bile, the liver's acrid yellow secretion, a man might vomit bile, a butchered animal might spill bile, let the bile not stain and spoil the meat. What shall be the fourth?

A beast has died, cut it open, and there in the left upper quadrant is a dark organ. We moderns would say the darkness is congealed blood, nothing more. The ancients would say the organ was filled with a liquid, a dark fluid. Let us call this black bile, the atrabilious humor, let us say that it resides in the spleen, opposite the liver, symmetry. The spleen's function they said was to collect black bile, *melaina kholē*, melancholy. The spleen is the seat of melancholy.

A splenic man has an excess of black bile. He is fretful, irritable, downhearted, his anatomic melancholy. And yet, Shakespeare's melancholy partakes also of lightness. Jaques speaks of "a melancholy of my own, compounded by many simples, extracted from many objects, and indeed the sundry contemplation of my travels, which, by often rumination, wraps me in a most humorous sadness." And in a book attributed for many centuries to Aristotle, the *Problems*, melancholy is the temperament of genius.

Burton's *Anatomy of Melancholy*, justly renowned, an encyclopedia of sadness and everything else, curious despondency, he writes of melancholy as a hedge against melancholy. Among the thousand strains of this multidirectional and often unraveling masterpiece, he tells how Hippocrates the physician one day found Democritus in a garden, writing and pacing, surrounded by the carcasses of dissected animals, seeking "to find out the seat of this black bile, or melancholy, whence it proceeds, and how it was engendered in men's bodies, to the intent he might better cure it in himself, and by his writings & observations teach others how to prevent and avoid it."

Austen, "Adieu to disappointment and spleen," the heroine anticipating a pleasant trip that should transport her from her troubles.

Baudelaire, his spleen, his poems of spleen, acrid tedium.

Nothing equals in length the limping days,
When under the heavy flakes of snow-covered years,
Ennui, fruit of dreary incuriosity,
Takes measure of immortality.

In prose his *Paris Spleen*, poems in prose; others came earlier, but his were the first of the great.

Baudelaire suffered manifold, and one of the forms his suffering took was a sense of being profoundly ill. And perhaps he was, so often he wrote his mother, I am sick, I am dying. A preoccupation, hypochondria, that ailment residing beneath the ribs, "*hypo*" + "*chondria*," splenetic excess. Syphilis was the disease that brought him down—an irony, no? For this disease too can enlarge the spleen.

A bacterium, a spirochete, invades the man and causes disease; or a man who is other-ill invites the bacterium to enter and to provide the corporeal expression of his inward malady. He was ill before syphilis, then contracted the spirochete, and syphilis became the form his illness took. His syphilis then is "pure art ... the creation of an evocative magic, containing at once the object and the subject, the world external to the artist and the artist himself."

Anthrax, a bacterium now of malevolent intent, was once called splenic fever, the modern bioterrorist thus recharges the ancient melancholy.

And for John Donne, "the ill affections of the *spleene*, complicate, and mingle themselves with every infirmitie of the body."

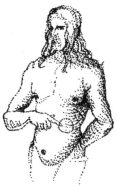

After Albrecht Dürer, "Self-portrait with the Yellow-Spot"

The splanchna, the viscera, in certain ancient sacrifices these were the parts reserved for the priests and select celebrants. There is even a verb, *splagchneuō*, to eat the innards of a victim after a sacrifice, also to prophesy from the innards.

The spleen may perform its destructive function to excess. The disease called immune thrombocytopenia purpura involves excessive destruction of platelets, the little cells of clotting. Chronic hemolytic anemia involves excessive destruction of red blood cells. One of the major therapies for both these conditions is an operation to remove the spleen, to destroy the destroyer, to unseat the seat of melancholy.

A motorcycle accident, a broken rib has lacerated the spleen, the spleen must be removed, an injured spleen must always be removed, excised, extirpated, surgical law, surgical logic, surgical emergency.

9. Marrow

BLOOD IS MADE IN THE BONE MARROW. OF ALL THE CAUSES OF anemia, the gravest are those caused by failure of the marrow.

The marrow is the great manufactory of blood cells. In leukemia, the production of blood cells is faulty, a single immature cell replicates itself without proper constraints and diverts the body's resources to its unchecked progeny. In aplastic anemia, the marrow stops production altogether. Certain chemicals, including alcohol and a number of powerful medicines, suppress the marrow's function and block cellular production.

The treatment of these diseases is drastic indeed. Unless some offending agent can be identified and removed, the only definitive therapy for leukemia or aplastic anemia is bone marrow transplantation. Chemotherapy, the most powerful of all chemotherapies, is administered to kill all the cells of the marrow, which is then replenished by infusions from a healthy donor.

A disease of the marrow cuts us to the very quick. In Ovid's *Metamorphoses*, Hercules is tricked into donning a poisoned shirt that burns horrifically, "dissolving his marrow." He prefers death. His friend Philoctetes, whose terrible wound forms the subject of dramas by each of the three great classical tragedians, answers the hero's plea and lights the pyre that burns him alive. Near the end of the same poem, the character of Pythagoras relates the belief that when the human spine has moldered in the grave, its marrow changes into a serpent. Sir Thomas Browne, the seventeenth-century physician and essayist, cites the same conceit in his great meditation on death, the *Hydriotaphia*.

The marrow is hidden from view, reached only by effort. To penetrate to the marrow is to reach the pith. Rabelais, physician and poet of sixteenth-century France, devotes his prologue to *Gargantua* to a discourse on marrow. Marrow is the dog's own truth:

> Did you ever see a dog coming upon some marrow bones? That is, as Plato says, Book 2 of *The Republic*, the most philosophic animal in the world. If seen one you have, you were able to note with what devotion he watches it, with what care he guards it, with what fervor he holds it, and with what prudence he starts on it, with what affection he breaks it, with what diligence he sucks it.

And simultaneously the poet's:

> After this example it behooves you to be wise enough to sniff out and assess these exquisite books, to be light footed in pursuit and bold in the encounter; then by careful reading and frequent meditation, break the bone and suck out the substantific marrow.

Pleasure and pith all together, the gnawing and the sweet reward.

For a person as for a book, the marrow is the innermost part, the core of one's being. "Be not wise in thine own eyes: fear the Lord, and depart from evil. / It shall be health to thy navel, and marrow to thy bones," says the Book of Proverbs. Who shall know our marrow? "For the word of God is quick, and powerful, and sharper than any two-edged sword, piercing even to the dividing asunder of soul and spirit, and of the joints and marrow, and is a discerner of the thoughts and intents of the heart."

Marrow, when eaten, is highly nutritious, rich in protein, fat, and vitamins. Early man may have begun to dine on animals not so much to obtain protein, which is readily available in the plant sources eaten by our vegetarian relatives the apes, as to obtain fat. They sought not flesh but marrow. The fossil records of early human encampments show animal bones split lengthwise, an action whose only rationale is to obtain the marrow within. Even recently, the archaeologist sees a boy of Kenya cracking a long bone from an antelope carcass to reach its marrow. In France, a smear of marrow on toast is a choice delicacy, and poached marrow graces croutons and sauces. In Italy, *ossobuco* makes for a tasty veal shank, but the best part is said to be the marrow, scooped from within the braised thigh-bone. In England, books of cookery and of medicine both have called the marrow delectable and wholesome since the fifteenth century at least. It is considered particularly easy to digest, appropriate for both babies and the infirm elderly.

The phrase rendered as "fat of the land" in the King James and Revised Standard Versions of the Bible is, in the Latin Vulgate, the "*medullam terrae*," the marrow of the land. The Hebrew word is "*chelev*," marrow.

The tastiest portion is the most suitable for feasting. Isaiah the prophet exalts his God, "And in this mountain shall the Lord of hosts make unto all people a feast of fat things, a feast of wines on the lees, of fat things full of marrow, of wines on the lees well refined." David the psalmist gives praise, "My soul shall be satisfied as with marrow and fatness; and my mouth shall praise thee with joyful lips." It might be noted that both these exultations celebrate the defiance of enemies; the marrow banquet is a victory feast, a glut and a gloat.

Feasting intersects sacrifice.

The marrow is the seat of love, love melts the marrow. When Virgil's Dido burns for Aeneas, love "inflames her soft marrow"; and when Shakespeare's Venus pleads with Adonis, "My flesh is soft and plump, my marrow burning." Catullus, who felt these things more than most men, recalls the support of his friend "when a raging flame scorched my marrow."

Conversely, the marrow is a man's strength. Hamlet the prince speaks of "the pith and marrow of our attribute," and Parolles the blowhard proclaims, in *All's Well that Ends Well*:

> To th' wars, my boy, to th' wars!
> He wears his honor in a box unseen,
> That hugs his kicky-wicky here at home,
> Spending his manly marrow in her arms,
> Which should sustain the bound and high curvet
> Of Mars's fiery steed.

The marrowbones are also the knees. To go down on your marrowbones is to pray.

Works of poetry often end in prose—or renunciation, or silence. The *Canterbury Tales* culminate in a prose sermon. Boccaccio repents of his fictions at the conclusion of the *Corbaccio*. Marlowe's Faustus pleads with Mephistopheles that he will burn his books, as Prospero says he will burn his books, as Virgil orders his *Aeneid* burned, and Kafka his manuscripts. Yeats, contemplating old age, writes or prays:

> God guard me from those thoughts men think
> In the mind alone;
> He that sings a lasting song
> Thinks in a marrow-bone;

And Rilke, having completed the *Duino Elegies* and the *Sonnets to Orpheus* in a cataclysm of creative production in 1922, age forty-seven, fell ill the next year. His disease was anemia and ultimately proved to be leukemia, a fatal affliction of the marrow. His blood and marrow turned against him in revolt. In 1925, less than a year before his death, he wrote these lines:

> Now may be time, that gods step out
> of inhabited things . . .
> and break down every wall
> in my house. New page.

10. Diseases of the Blood

TO THE PATIENT, DISEASES OF THE BLOOD SEEM PARTICULARLY menacing. The mind turns first to leukemia, among the most terrifying of all diseases. Multiple myeloma, refractory anemia, myelodysplasia—even their names inspire fear.

Other organs also have special meaning, whether healthy or diseased. The heart, liver, and brain seem to evoke the greatest emotional charges—dating at least to the time of Galen, when these three corresponded to the three pneumas; the Vital, Natural, and Psychic. For Shakespeare, these three were the body's "sovereign thrones." Diseases in these organs bring a heightened reaction, compared with those, say, of the kidneys or the intestines. Medical authors, since antiquity, have contended which of the three is the seat of the soul, or whether each is home to a department of the tripartite soul, but only these three, never the lungs, the stomach, the elbow. These latter hold a secondary position, a lower or debased status. In contemporary times, only the organs of sexuality contend for primacy.

Heart attack—my heart has been attacked, I will never be the same, my life is changed, changed utterly. The term misstates what actually happens when the heart is damaged. *Myocardial infarction,* or the older *coronary thrombosis,* renders in technical pathological language the same fearful image. A man has chest pain, he comes to the hospital, the doctor interprets the electrocardiogram, performs blood tests—you are having a heart attack, an artery to the heart has closed down, a portion of the heart is dying. Who could ever be the same?

The treatment, a generation ago, was rest and little more. When President Eisenhower suffered a heart attack in his third year of office, age sixty-four, the doctors ordered him to bed and commanded rest for two months. Heart disease deactivated the mighty general, took him out of commission, emasculated him to a degree. Heart attack then meant a subsequent life as an invalid. The President's unexpectedly vigorous recovery lent significant strength to his successful re-election campaign the following year.

A modern heart attack is something quite different. Even the traditional myocardial infarction is eminently treatable. Moreover, the diagnostic blood test used most widely today, called troponin, is so sensitive that it routinely detects even the slightest damage to the heart. Medicine has yet to find a word for these incidents of minor, often trivial damage to the heart. The doctors speak among themselves of a "troponin leak"—he spilled some troponin—an affectionate and trivializing nickname. How cute, a little leak, a bit of a spill, like coffee sloshing over the brim; well anyway there's a saucer. What shall they tell the patient? Your heart had a little damage, but don't worry, it's minor, I'm sure you'll be okay. Doctor did I have a heart attack? Well, yes, sort of, it is a kind of heart attack, a little one, you'll just have to take some medicine. The physicians struggle to minimize what the patient has learned as the most dramatic of all illness events. They are already translating the illness into action plans; this one can be managed medically, merely medically. The patient requires medicines but not surgery, nor the surgical surrogate now called percutaneous coronary intervention that includes angioplasty (balloon procedure), rotational atherectomy (another affectionate nickname, "Roto-Rooter"), and stent. The only precise medical term, a non-ST elevation myocardial infarction (non-STEMI), is so technically jargonized as to be incomprehensible except within an internal cardiology discourse. Never could "non-STEMI" mean anything to a patient.

The patient's term refers to something he feels, a heart attack, my heart and life are under attack. The doctors' older terms translate the event into something they see, or rather would see, under the microscope—and, since we are talking of hearts, to see a heart under the microscope is to examine the results of an autopsy, to speak of an infarction is to imagine that the patient has died and that his tissues are under postmortem scrutiny. The doctors' newer term refers to something they see on the electrocardiogram: the ST portion of the tracing has moved a certain way. Their newest concept, the troponin leak, has yet to find a dignified name.

The liver is the second of the major organs without which none may survive. Nature has provided most organs in pairs, the eyes, the ears, lungs, kidneys, adrenal glands, breasts, ovaries, testes, the arms and legs, the two lobes of the thyroid. To lose one of the pairs is most unfortunate but not catastrophic, not fatal, none is indispensable. The strange unpaired organs of the abdomen are the liver, in the right upper portion, and the spleen, in the left upper portion, and so unusual is the occurrence of such asymmetry that the ancient physiologists struggled to assign them a symmetry, either in anatomy or function. Aristotle, for example, waffled as to whether the liver and spleen constituted one organ or two. Physicians for millennia have conceived the liver as the organ that makes blood, and what then shall the spleen do? Perhaps it cleans the blood or destroys old blood, and indeed in these splenic conjectures the ancients were mainly right.

The pancreas, in the middle, was so unknowable that its peculiar name broaches on mysticism, "*pan-kreas*," all-flesh.

Liver disease today means three main things. First is infectious hepatitis, described with great clinical accuracy in all the ancient writings, jaundice, the eyes and skin have turned an insidious shade of bilious yellow. The ancients contracted hepatitis by ingesting contaminated food or by the bites of certain infected mosquitoes, and so too may the moderns, but the hepatitis that looms larger today is transmitted by sexual contact and intravenous (or intranasal) drug use—the patient brought it upon himself, he is blamable and not merely hapless. Blamable, too, is the patient with alcoholic cirrhosis; he drank himself to death, bloated and jaundiced, a failed human being. Cancer, as well, commonly strikes the liver, and while primary cancers of the liver occur mainly in people with pre-existing liver disease, that is in those already condemned by their putatively self-induced cirrhosis, secondary or metastatic tumors of the liver are the all-too-common omens of fatal cancer. A cancer that has traveled to the liver cannot be cured, the doctor tells the patient of a liver metastasis, the doctor speaks hopefully of some promising chemotherapy, the patient believes it not, the patient knows he is to die.

Moses Maimonides: "In the health of the liver lies our livelihood, as Galen has also said." The belief persists in contemporary France, where the liver commands special valence as the key to health and disease.

Brain disease has meant two main things: madness and epilepsy. Not always was it clear that these arose from the brain. Many eminent authorities questioned whether the brain did anything at all, or did anything more important than to process input from the sensory organs, or to produce phlegm. (Aristotle wrote that the brain's main function was to moderate the heat of the heart and to cool the blood.) In contrast, the Hippocratic text *On the Sacred Disease* presents one of the seminal moments in medical history, arguing that epilepsy was not a divine visitation or curse but a disease of the brain akin to any other disease. The author had observed an epileptic seizure in a goat with putrefaction (infection) of the brain. The brain is a body part among others, an exceptional one, but nowise supernatural.

To a modern, epilepsy has lost much of its terror and its mystery—pills work, most of the time, no one would ever know. Madness goes by other names: depression, ubiquitous, treatable; bipolar disorder, awful but awe-inspiring, perhaps a gift. Schizophrenia, the broken mind, strikes the teenager and young adult, no adult past that age need fear developing it. The brain disease that terrifies the modern is dementia, to become dementified, to lose the *mens*, the mind. A century ago the disease one feared most was tuberculosis, consumption; a generation ago, cancer; but now it is dementia that reigns supreme, a grim, gray and hideous god who wields his scepter like a coarse-hewn club, ready to smite the brain and mind. Any fifty-year-old has felt his insinuating warning, a forgotten name here, a lost fact there, is this ordinary forgetfulness or a sign of early Alzheimer's disease, Oh God may it not be Alzheimer's. The modern term disguises the fact but no one is fooled, dementia is the same, second childishness and mere oblivion, sans teeth, sans eyes, sans taste, sans everything.

In one of ancient Rome's darkest hours, when Hannibal threatened the city with destruction after the Battle of Lake Trasimene (217 BCE), the republic dedicated two shrines to Mens, the personification of mind. Mens is the defense against annihilation.

Diseases of the blood somehow stand apart. One of the greatest themes in all of medicine is the contest between two very different concepts of disease. Does disease constitute a global imbalance of the body's properties and energies, or rather an affliction of a body part or organ? The first idea, which one might call the humoral theory, predominates in the medical philosophies of China, India, Greece, Rome, Europe, and the Arabic-speaking world up to the eighteenth century. In these worldviews, the body and indeed all of nature consist in the balance of elements. Disease consists in their imbalance. This is the central idea in yin-yang, in the three-humor system of Ayurvedic medicine, and in the four-humor system of the Greco-Roman-Arabic tradition.

The second, competing idea, which one might call organ-based pathology, occurs in early medicine but first predominates during the Industrial Revolution. It is a theory of parts. Its first great exponent is Giovanni Battista Morgagni, whose magnum opus *On the Sites and Causes of Diseases* (1761) demonstrates the relation between specific diseases and specific abnormalities found in specific organs on autopsy. Jaundice, previously conceived as an overabundance of the bilious humor, is instead the result of a diseased liver. By the time two generations had passed, the locus of disease is not the organ but a tissue within the organ; thus Marie François Xavier Bichat, who describes the microscopic findings in diseased organs in his *Treatise on Membranes* (1800). Two generations more, and the focus turns from the tissue to the cell in the lectures of the physician and anthropologist Rudolf Virchow, whose *Cellular Pathology as Based upon Physiological and Pathological Histology* appears in 1858. The twentieth century zooms in even closer, as Linus Pauling, twice a Nobel laureate, announces that sickle-cell disease resides in an abnormal molecule (1949). Now the twenty-first century focuses closer still—the disease may be a gene, a faulty blueprint.

Where stands blood disease? Is blood an organ? Like the liver and the heart, blood possesses a specific identity—one can say, this is blood and this is not—and serves specific functions. Unlike these organs, however, blood knows no specific locus in the body. Blood is everywhere, global. The blood is not flesh. Is blood then a humor? In Greco-Roman-Arabic medicine, yes: this tradition counts blood as one of the four humors, or vital fluids, but one that generally plays a subsidiary role to bile and phlegm, the more prominent humoral actors. Ayurvedic medicine also expresses ambivalence as to whether blood should be a humor or not. The three classical Indian humors are *vāta* (wind/breath/air), *pitta* (bile/fire), and *kapha* (phlegm/mucus/water). Whether *pāndu* (blood) should be a fourth was never decided.

Diseases of the blood thus participate in both concepts, a humoral disease and an organ-based pathology. Blood is the body's place that knows no place, knowing every place. Blood is the conveyor of *pneuma*, *arwah*, *spiritus*, breath, of vital energy, of life itself. To lose blood is to die.

We speak even now of blood poisoning. The modern concept is septicemia, a spread of bacterial infection to the blood itself, a severe condition that causes death in one of five cases. The underlying concept, not far from the modern picture, is contamination of the blood, the blood is poisoned, the blood is sullied. A foreign and malevolent substance enters the body, a barbarous organism invades the body, the worm, the demon, the hex, it disseminates its evil everywhere throughout the body, no part shall be spared. We all have had infections, we all know that if an infection spreads to the blood we are in serious trouble, we labor to control the infection locally to prevent its spreading globally. A miniature quarantine, a containment, cast out the stranger he may bear pestilence, if thy hand offend thee cut it off. A farmer drains pus with his pocketknife, he drains it outward lest it spread inward, sound clinical practice, he calls his abscess proud flesh.

Bad blood is faithlessness, a violation of trust. *Bad blood between us*, an abrogation, the Hatfields and the McCoys, a blood feud, never to be reconciled. The opposite is blood brothers, ever trusted, eternally bound.

Aceldama is the Field of Blood. Judas cast back the thirty pieces of silver before he hanged himself, the chief priests would not take them up, blood money, the price of blood.

With it they bought the potter's field, Aceldama, to bury strangers in.

Spilt blood, blood curse, the one begets the other. Cain spills his brother's blood, suffers the curse of God, which is the curse of the earth, "which hath opened her mouth to receive thy brother's blood from thy hand." God is speaking. The blood of Abel, the curse of Cain, blood vengeance, "That upon you may come all the righteous blood shed upon the earth, from the blood of righteous Abel unto the blood of Zacharias son of Barachias, whom ye slew between the temple and the altar."

The Erinyes, the Furies, the Avengers, these daughters of Earth sprang from the blood of the mutilated Uranus.

Blood vengeance intersects disease. In Aeschylus's *The Libation Bearers*, the middle drama of the Oresteia trilogy, the Chorus sings of the blood curse on the house of Atreus, the father has killed the daughter, the wife has killed the husband, the son has killed the mother, and spilt blood begets disease that infects the guilty. The victim's blood stains and penetrates the murder, it corrodes and corrupts his own blood, he putrefies, he bears disease, he breeds disease that none may allay. Blood disease is uniquely a corruption, something is rotten, the patient might contaminate another, though in medical fact he cannot. Blood disease is blood guilt, blood disease reenacts the buried, ancient drama in which sick blood stems from *nefas*, blasphemy.

Blood-stained, sickened Orestes sought Apollo, he supplicated the god, he came to trial, the goddess Athena cast the vote that acquitted the man and decided his fate. The blood-sick modern seeks the physician, but who could equal the ancient forgiveness, and who could transform the avenging Erinyes into the peace-giving Eumenides? The physician pledged the Hippocratic Oath, I swear by Apollo the physician, but modern sentiments have extirpated the god, he may not here remain.

Some diseases, known for centuries, have become familiar. Tuberculosis can be a terrible disease, but rarely is it terrifying; a man coughs blood, ah, the old familiar strikes, I know what is happening and what is to come, my life shall play itself out, I am to be consumed but not ravaged. Diseases newly recognized may or may not be quickly tamed. Thus osteoporosis, a new disease, should not incite terror in the newly diagnosed patient. There is a treatment, there is a pill, and indeed this condition became known as a disease only when there arrived a medicine to treat it, the pill fathers the diagnosis. Ditto hypercholesterolemia, ditto irritable bladder, ditto athlete's foot. Even HIV/AIDS, a new disease, was terrifying in its first decades but placable in its latter years. Yet leukemia, a new disease first recognized in the early twentieth century, has never been tamed and always incites terror. The condition that the nineteenth century called splenic anemia proved to be a cancer of the white blood cells, a blood cancer, and what could be more dire than that?

All leukemias are not the same. Chronic lymphocytic leukemia runs a slow and gradual course, so bland that it rarely requires treatment in the first five or ten years after diagnosis. Some, indeed, have questioned whether it should be called leukemia at all, pointing out the harmful consequences of such a frightful label. Chronic myelocytic leukemia runs a tougher course but remains manageable. In contrast, the acute leukemias are rapid and devastating, causing death within a few weeks if not treated, and the treatments themselves demand much and often prove fatal. No patient ever hears the word leukemia without expecting death. One would have to reach back to the Black Death of fourteenth-century Europe, or the plague of seventeenth-century London, to find accounts of a diagnosis with such immediately devastating psychological consequences.

A disease of the blood is like no other, no where, everywhere, offering no line to stake a defense, no bulwark, no battlement, the horde has forced the city, the walls are down, a bloodthirsty multitude, pillage, rapine, the gig is up, the city is fallen, the king is slain, and I am going to die.

11. Anemia World

IN THE DEVELOPED WORLD, OR WHAT MIGHT BETTER BE called the materially developed world, anemia is important only insofar as it signifies something else. Anemia might mean cancer, anemia might mean leukemia or one of its precursors. Anemia in itself infrequently makes one sick.

In many countries of Africa, Latin America, and South Asia, however, anemia means something different altogether. There, anemia makes people sick. Worldwide, anemia is a major cause of death, especially in children and women. Women with anemia bear weakened children and are more susceptible to death during childbirth. Anemia saps children of their full capacity for physical and intellectual growth, and adults of their full capacity for work.

How many people? The World Health Organization (WHO) estimates that two billion people suffer from anemia, up to a third of the world's population. A recent study in Côte d'Ivoire found that about half the children and adult women had anemia.

One might well question what these figures mean. They are defined, as good modern statistics are, in terms of deviance from numerical norms. This begs the question of *which* norm. In developed countries, the normal hemoglobin level in men is 14–18 g/dL. Most healthy men fall within this range. WHO defines anemia, for its purposes, as hemoglobin less than 12 g/dL. No one doubts that a man with a hemoglobin level of 8 g/dL will feel the effects of his anemia. But a man with hemoglobin 11 g/dL will probably feel well and work well. That is, his statistical deviance is not harmful. Is he anemic? He certainly is not pale. He does not feel sick. He *is* not sick.

In the developing world, the three main causes of anemia are dietary iron deficiency, infestation with intestinal worms, and infection with malaria. Inadequate dietary intake accounts for about half the world's anemia. Humans seem to require more iron in their diet than most diets provide. This is all the more true of women, who require more iron than men but for whom many cultures restrict access to meat. Why might humans need so much iron in their diets? Most likely we evolved in an environment in which dietary iron was plentiful—which basically means that our evolutionary ancestors ate a lot of meat. (Alternately, we might have once been better at absorbing small amounts of iron from our then diverse foodstuffs.) In either case, iron deficiency is yet another of the compromises of civilization. For the diet of early civilization, based heavily on such agricultural grains as wheat, barley, maize, and rice, provides ample calories to support a large population but rather little iron. Anemia seems to have occurred infrequently among hunting societies but commonly among early farmers, in whom the prevalence approached fifty percent. (Many diseases, too, first appear in humans in the early days of civilization, when tuberculosis crossed over from cattle, influenza from poultry, and measles from dogs, as HIV was later to cross over from apes.)

Iron deficiency, it appears, is a disease of civilization, a compromise of the agricultural revolution. Not exactly a disease of surfeit, such as modern-day diabetes, obesity, and ischemic heart disease—iron deficiency arose in populations when a surfeit of calories from carbohydrates outpaced the available supply of iron. It is easily overcome by those with access to meat-rich diets, iron-enriched foods, or iron sup-

plement tablets—in other words, to citizens of the prosper-
ous nations—but not by the world's other peoples. For modern humans, iron sufficiency is a condition of wealth, iron
deficiency of poverty.

Intestinal worms, or helminths, which affect some two
billion people worldwide, cause anemia in three main ways.
Hookworm and schistosoma, the most important of the parasitic worms, live in the human intestine where they consume
nutrients, induce bleeding, and suck blood. They too first
appeared in the human archaeologic record during the period
of early civilization. In some instances, for example the round-
worm ascara, the parasite probably crossed from pigs to humans
at a time when the domestication of animals brought unprece-
dented proximity between the two species. In others, for example the flatworm schistosoma, the conditions of agriculture
created major breeding grounds for a hitherto minor organism.

Schistosomiasis, infecting some 200 million people
worldwide, warrants particular attention. It is carried by various snails that live in the standing waters of ponds, irrigation
ditches, and rice paddies. Humans contract the infection
when they wade, swim, or bathe in such water. The parasite
can then affect nearly every organ in the body. The huge dis-
tended abdomens that give the disease its moniker "big
belly" result from damage to the liver.

Somber news: a pill that costs about twenty cents will
eliminate schistosoma infection about ninety-five percent
of the time. For the next most important infection, hookworm, treatment costs about two cents. A Coke costs a dol-
lar, enough to treat fifty children with hookworm.

Malaria, the foremost parasitic disease of planet Earth, is
the third major cause of anemia among its human denizens.
Its essential features have been recognized for thousands of

years. Malaria tends to cause a particular pattern of fever that occurs every three days, or every four days, quite different from the daily spikes of most febrile illnesses. Tertian and quartan fevers feature prominently in the Hippocratic, Ayurvedic, and Chinese texts, and indeed their periodicity was easy to extrapolate into statements about the periodicity of illness in general, their specific temporal outlines, their tendency to culminate in a dramatic and singular crisis that portended death or cure. A template of relapsing fever dominated medical thinking for centuries.

Dante, about to descend to the lowest circles of Hell, compares himself to one nearing the recrudescence of quartan fever, malaria, his nails already pale, trembling at the mere sight of shadow.

Malaria, *mal-aria*, bad air, evil air. The word parallels other Italian semantic constructions designating evil: thus *malocchio*, the evil eye. In his 1881 short story "Malaria," the Sicilian Giovanni Verga makes no distinction between the noxious air of low-lying places and the disease it seemed to cause.

The disease occurred near swampy areas. Was there some toxic miasma that emanated from such places? Were they poisonous, the shimmering mists that arose from fens and quagmires? The Hippocratic text *Humors* speaks of certain diseases that stem from the smells of slime and marshes. Did some invisible creature breed there? Thus Marcus Terentius Varro, a Roman author of the first century BCE: "Avoid marshy places . . . because there grow certain minute, invisible animals that are carried through the air, enter the body through the mouth and the nose, and cause difficult diseases." The Romans, of course, were master drainers of swamps.

The Incans understood that a certain bark, from the cinchona tree, could successfully treat fever. The active ingredient was quinine, whose derivatives are still effective therapies for malaria. The English distrusted a putative medicine imported from Spanish colonies; the Peruvian bark was Jesuit powder, maybe a treacherous poison. The innovative therapy, however, eventually caught on. Patients soon took cinchona for any fever, time passed, millions of doses, and the drug no longer worked. The same pattern—innovative antimicrobial therapy, cautious use, widespread use, overuse, resistance, ineffectiveness—was later to repeat itself many times, for newer antimalarials, for penicillin, and for a host of other therapies.

In the late nineteenth century, stimulated by colonial interests in warm regions as much as by the spirit of scientific inquiry, medicine solved the essential riddle. Malaria is an infectious disease, transmitted by the bite of a certain genus of mosquito, *Anopheles*, that harbors a complex one-celled organism called *Plasmodium*. The disease occurs near swamps because there the mosquitoes breed and live. Drain the swamps, kill the mosquitoes, and malaria will disappear. And so it did, or almost did, in North America and Europe. Nobel Prizes earned and received.

The periodicity of fever is not a universal property of disease in general but rather the specific result of the *Plasmodium* life cycle. An infected female mosquito bites a person and injects saliva contaminated with *Plasmodium* cysts. These enter the human red blood cells, multiply, and cause the cell to rupture, releasing further *Plasmodium* particles. These bursts occur synchronously, accounting for the periodic fevers.

Malaria kills some million children a year, most of them in Africa. About half the world's population lives in areas endemic for malaria, and clinical malaria strikes some 350–500 million people each year, perhaps one in twelve of all the world's people.

For adults, the acute bouts of fever are most unpleasant and sometimes fatal, but not automatically worse than such commonplace Western diseases as influenza. From the perspective of anemia, the central point is that the infected red blood cells burst. Malaria causes chronic anemia by bursting the red blood cells. A person chronically infected with malaria is chronically tired, enfeebled, debilitated, hobbled, shackled. Little gets done.

The countries with the highest rates of malaria, above all those in Africa, are those with the lowest per capita incomes and the lowest rates of economic development. Many have argued that malaria is a major cause of underdevelopment both at the personal and national levels. One study concludes that malaria is responsible for a reduction in economic growth estimated at 1.3 percent per annum in the countries most affected.

Such an explanation strengthens the resolve to combat malaria and assuages the liberal conscience. The poor countries must be impoverished by malaria; their material poverty has a material cause. These recall the arguments of the past, that people in warm countries were naturally torpid and lazy, while those in cold lands were naturally vigorous and energetic. They admire us, they would be like us, would emulate us—they don't because they can't.

One can only wonder whether malaria, like iron deficiency and the helminth infections, could be a disease of civilization. Malaria probably predates civilization, but widespread malaria becomes most possible when farmers clear forests, irrigate fields, collect water, and build cisterns. These form the expanded habitats of the *Anopheles* mosquito, and here the disease expands. In African prehistory, the phenomenon took place during the Neolithic Era, when early horticulturists migrated south into equatorial regions. The same phenomenon occurs in contemporary times, as malaria increases in such tropical areas as the Amazon during the initial phases of the frontier.

Four species of *Plasmodium* infect humans: *P. malariae, P. ovale, P. vivax*, and *P. falciparum*. Of these, the last is deadliest by far. *Falciparum* malaria, the main form in Africa, is so named because the organism resembles a sickle, in Latin "*falx*." And why, again, do we speak of sickles? Crescent malaria would have done just as well to describe the parasite's shape. But here again the sickle rears its head, makes itself known, the reaper, the slayer, malevolent harvest.

Two hereditary conditions, thalassemia trait and sickle-cell trait, help defend against malaria but also can cause mild anemia. Thus, malaria contributes to African anemia by an additional, backdoor mechanism, providing evolutionary pressure to accept mild anemia in exchange for partial malaria resistance.

Malaria once reigned in the United States as well, although temperate climates were never so hospitable to *Anopheles* as were subtropical and tropical neighbors. Now, most cases of malaria in North America occur in travelers who contracted the disease overseas. Mosquito control measures eliminated malaria from the continent—or did they? As recently as 2003, eight persons developed malaria within the United States, presumably bitten by infected mosquitoes. Malaria is not gone from here but merely sleeps. The *Anopheles* mosquito could be found, the *Plasmodium* parasite could be found, but what keeps them at bay is a social infrastructure. And if the infrastructure were compromised? Collapsed? And if the swamps came back?

An attack of malaria weakens a man, an attack of malaria strengthens a man, because he is better able to resist future infections. To be a carrier of sickle-cell anemia, remember, also conveys partial resistance to malaria. And if the swamps return, and if some new breed of *Plasmodium* outwits our drugs, who shall better resist the onslaught: the well-fed but disease-naïve American, or the anemic, disease-experienced African? Who then shall be weak, and who shall be strong?

IV. TREATMENT /
WHAT WOULD THEY DO TO ME?

The foremost purpose of Medicine is to reduce suffering. The physician's therapeutic tools—a pill, an operation, a special kind of talk—all aim toward this goal. Each age defines its therapies in terms of its own understanding of the body and the world, declaring them both rational and verified. One rejects all other explanations as superstitious or ignorant. But even the most effective treatments often derive from an earlier age's reason, later castigated by subsequent eras as unreason.

12. Iron

Iron, nowadays an eminently rational treatment for anemia, begins its therapeutic life in mythology, alchemy, and magic. Like Newton's theory of gravitation, stimulated in large part by his ten-year study of alchemy; like Copernicus's concept of heliocentric orbits, stirred by images of Neoplatonic forms and Hermetic circles; like Kekulé's discovery of the benzene ring, inspired by a dream, canonical science often starts somewhere far from the laboratory.

Iron, a metal, the most abundant element on earth, plays a central role in one of life's great organic dramas. Nearly all living cells, be they plant or animal, require oxygen. The great life formula, oxygen + glucose $\rightarrow$ carbon dioxide + water + energy, requires that oxygen be available everywhere throughout the organism. (It mimics fire, which follows the same essential steps to yield heat, light, and flame.) The smallest creatures, such as bacteria and amoebas, accomplish this essential distribution by simple diffusion of the gas from the outer environment. Larger creatures, including amphibians, reptiles, birds, fish, and mammals, require an oxygen-transport system. They have evolved a unique molecule, hemoglobin, to carry the oxygen, and a unique conveyance, blood, to distribute the hemoglobin throughout the body.

The core of the hemoglobin molecule, and hence the core of blood itself, is iron. Each hemoglobin molecule cradles four atoms of this stout metal, and each atom can bind and release an atom of oxygen. In another of the infinite macrocosm–microcosm correspondences that would so fascinate the Renaissance, the iron at the core of planet Earth is the iron at the core of human blood.

The commonest cause of anemia in modern humans is insufficient dietary iron. (Before agriculture radically changed human diets for all time, prehistoric man had ample access to iron, mainly from meat, and rarely developed anemia.) Although the metal is ubiquitous, people do not eat stones, and if they did they could not absorb, or not very well, the mineral form of iron. Many plant foods, too, contain iron, but also in a form that the human digestive tract cannot absorb efficiently. Animal flesh, on the other hand, contains abundant iron, and in a highly usable ("bioavailable") form called myoglobin. It is myoglobin that gives meat its red color, and red meats provide more iron than pale meats.

Eating or drinking blood might also provide dietary iron, but this practice is taboo in most cultures. Kosher law forbids it, and so does Islamic dietary law (*halāl*). A few societies, such as the Berbers, the Mongols, and the Masai, all herdsmen, endorse the drinking of blood. Most modern Americans would find doing so disgusting, a physiologic expression of taboo, and the modern European eats such stuff as *Blutwurst* (blood sausage) or black pudding (made of congealed blood) only sparingly, if at all, a form of gustatory reminiscence. The maybe sturdier palate of Mexican cuisine considers *jugo de carne*, a broth of blood and juices extracted from lightly cooked beef, a restorative soup, useful in treating anemia. Drinking blood, although it would be dietetically efficient, occurs primarily in ritual: the triumphant warrior on the one hand, the Eucharist celebrant on the other.

There was a rumor, oft repeated and oft disputed, that the Athenian statesman Themistocles committed suicide by drinking the blood of a bull, which caused instant death.

Voltaire specifically rejects the story, noting that he often saw peasants drinking cow's blood without ill effect, and he himself had tried the experiment.

Modern breakfast cereals boast of being *fortified* with iron, the metal makes them strong, the metal makes you strong too, buy me, eat me up. To call iron a supplement or additive would weaken the pitch considerably.

Aside from foods, certain mineral waters might provide a source of iron. Springs have been associated with healing since prehistoric times. Such sites as Grisy in France, Forlì in Italy, and Saint Moritz in Switzerland have known sacred healing cults since the Neolithic and Bronze Ages. Elsewhere nymphs, naiads, water sprites, and other demigods have sanctified and vivified springs. Mineral springs—those in which the waters have a particularly high mineral content—have often been viewed as especially healthful. The minerals in question may be sulfur, most of all, but also calcium, sodium, magnesium, potassium—and iron. So-called chalybeate waters (named after the Chalybes, a people of Asia Minor known for the working of iron) were rich in iron and might be taken medicinally. Visiting a mineral spring, bath, or spa, of course, could mean not only bathing in the healthful waters but drinking them; thus "taking the waters" in Jane Austen's eighteenth-century Bath, thus the Pump Room.

While mineral waters might have been considered healthful, be the reason sacred or profane, ancient authors did not advocate iron-rich waters specifically. The first to do so was the Persian physician Ibn Sīnā (Avicenna), who wrote that "waters which contain metallic substances are generally injurious. Some may however be of considerable value, i.e., water with iron strengthens the internal organs, prevents stomach trouble and stimulates the appetite." Moreover, he continues in a later passage, "Ferruginous waters are beneficial for the stomach and spleen. . . . Aerated waters, ferruginous and saline waters are beneficial for diseases depending on coldness and moisture, for pains in the joints, for podagra. They benefit relaxed persons, asthma, renal disease, carbuncles, ulcers. They are very beneficial in case of fracture."

Finally, the physician might prescribe iron in the form of a medicine. Ayurvedic practitioners generally advocated therapies based on herbs, sometimes on minerals. The ancient *Suśruta Samhitā*, for example, classified minerals as one of the thirty-seven groups of drugs, naming tin, lead, copper, silver, gold, and iron. As a group, these were used for worms, heart diseases, urinary disorders, and anemia. Iron, in particular, was recommended for severe pallor—although, lest this be heralded as an early discovery of iron-deficiency anemia, the text also recommends ghee (clarified butter), turmeric, and various herbs suspended in cow's urine as treatments for related conditions.

In Zanzibar, a traditional treatment for anemia is *chomwe*, a mixture of iron filings and herbal medicines. Although persons taking *chomwe* draw no parallels with iron tablets, also available on the island, the name probably stems from *chuma*, the Swahili word for iron.

Greek and Roman physicians prescribed mineral drugs occasionally but iron seldom. Dioscorides Pedanius, a Greek physician serving in the Roman army who authored the definitive first-century pharmacopoeia *Materia Medica*, recommends drinking a concoction of iron rust to prevent pregnancy and to treat heavy menses, as well as various digestive ailments. Topical preparations are suggested to treat skin conditions. He makes no connection with anemia or pallor. Arabic medicine, as we have seen, recommended ferrous mineral waters but not specifically ferrous drugs.

★   ★   ★

Iron has always touched on magic. The earliest examples of worked iron derived from meteorites, stones that fell from heaven. They date from the third millennium BCE. Moreover, the smithy is a place of magic, where fire and human skill meet to effect transformation. A stone lump, metamorphosis, a spearhead, a scythe; inert matter becomes a tool, a weapon, agency. The Cyclopes, monstrous giants, forge the thunderbolts of Zeus. Their master Hephaestus, the Greek god of the smithy, is a paradox—an underground fire god, he lives in darkness, he lives by flame, a lame craftsman, a pitiable hero, wedded to the goddess of love who proffers him no love but only scorn. Aphrodite bears him no children. Yet in his home, under the volcano Etna, he creates marvels in metal, the armor of Achilles, the necklace of Harmonia, and perhaps he creates even life, Pandora, the first or quintessential woman, or near-life, Talos, the artificial bronze man who guarded Crete.

The Telchines, demigods of Rhodes, were skilled in metal and in magic, dangerous, mischievous, not to be trusted. In one account they were the first to work metal, in another the first to make images of the gods; in a third they craft the sickle that Kronos wields to castrate his father, Uranus; and in a fourth they forge the trident of Poseidon. Others say the first smiths were the Dactyls, dwarfs of Crete, workmen of Hephaestus, sorcerers and wizards.

The dwarfs of Norse mythology too are smiths, they forge the hammer of Thor and the necklace of Freya, herself a sorceress of dubious practice. Alberich the dwarf crafts the ring that casts the fate and downfall of the gods. The gnomes, too, were workers in metal, masters of trickery, endowed with magic; the gods can coax or outwit but never fully dominate them. Iron is an underworld power, brought up from under the earth, animated by fire.

The world's oldest known mine, at Bomvu Ridge in the Ngwenya Mountains of Swaziland, dates to some 42,000 years ago. There, Paleolithic humans dug for iron. What they sought, however, was not workable metal but *pigment*. The purpose of the mine, an enormous undertaking for people using stone tools, was to provide the red colors with which our ancestors painted both rock walls and themselves. Iron oxide is hematite, the bloodlike stone, red ocher, its color is red. *Bomvu* is the Zulu word for red.

Even older, but probably found rather than mined, were the lumps of iron oxide called rock ocher. The oldest known symbolic object in human history, found in the Blombos Cave near the southernmost tip of Africa, is an ocher plaque incised with an abstract geometric design. It dates to some 70,000 years ago.

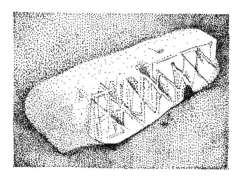

By contrast, the oldest cave paintings of Europe, also drawn or colored with ocher, date to some 30,000 years ago.

The use of red ocher, presumably for decoration and body painting, provides one of the oldest known human instances of symbolic expression, and thus one of modern humanity's earliest signatures. Paleoanthropologists date the behavior to the Middle Stone Age and report that the earliest known examples of ground ocher, found in the Kapthurin Formation in Kenya, were made over 285,000 years ago.

Red ocher, iron oxide, also provided the main red pigment in Egyptian and Roman painting—although the really good stuff, far more costly, was realgar (arsenic disulfide), from Lower Nubia or Solfatara near Naples, and cinnabar (mercuric sulfide), from Almaden in Spain. In the Americas, people surrounding the Great Lakes in the first millennium BCE developed a distinctive burial practice, rubbing ocher into the bare bones of the dead and sprinkling it over their grave goods, for which archaeologists have named theirs the Red Ocher Culture.

Iron too confers worldly power. Prehistory traces a sequence from the Stone Age to the Bronze Age and finally to the Iron Age, the latest and greatest of civilization's advances. Whatever people masters the new advanced technology conquers its neighbors and reigns supreme, at least for a while. As we all learned in grade school, the first to master iron technology were the Hittites, founders of the first Indo-European culture, whose empire spread from Asia Minor to dominate the Middle East in the second millennium BCE. The Dorian invaders who swept out of northwest Greece around 1100 BCE wielded iron swords, dealing the death-blow to the Mycenaean civilization of the late Bronze Age. The Egyptians, in contrast, had no iron tools or weapons until the eighth century BCE. They called iron *ba-n-pet*, the metal from heaven, it fell from the sky, meteorite.

In Indo-European, the common ancestor of most of the languages of Europe, western and southwestern Asia, and the northern Indian subcontinent, the root for the modern word "iron" is *eis*, "holy." Already by the sixth millennium BCE, language held iron to be sacred—perhaps because it came from the sky, perhaps because it was used for sacred purposes.

A material view of world history asserts that each new instrumentality, each new means of domination, carries humankind forward, but so too it may carry us backward. So the ancients counted the *descent* from the Golden Age, when Kronos ruled an ever youthful race of men, "untouched by work or sorrow," to the Silver, Bronze, and finally the Iron Ages. The Greek mythological view of history considers the last and present age to be the worst of times, a sequence not of incremental progress but of decremental loss of piety, health, and benevolence. For Hesiod, writing approximately in 700 BCE,

> For now is the race of iron. By day men
> Labor ceaselessly, wretchedly, while by night
> They meet their ruin.

Iron is power, iron too is cold, violent, and bloodthirsty. Men first used iron for jewelry, ornament, and the ritual objects of worship. It was rare then, sacred matter. The subsequent master use was weaponry, manufactured and profane. Peaceful uses—the scythe, the cooking pot, the plow—arrived later still.

Ovid traces the same descent from the Golden Age. But his Iron Age is not the poet's present. Rather, having misbegotten war, money, and a thousand other evils on earth and in heaven, the Age of Iron invokes the wrath of Zeus, who sends the flood that drowns all human life, sparing only Deucalion and Pyrrha, the Greek Noah and his wife. Elderly, pious, and reverent, only they survive to create a new race of humans from stones they throw over their shoulders, and this race is our own. For the poet,

> Hence we are the stock of hardness, and our toil
> Gives testimony to the origin of our birth.

The sole survivors of the Age of Iron are our own ancestral parents, and we are creatures made from stones.

John Donne goes a step further: "Our age was Iron, and rusty too."

Ancient Persian mythology referred to four ages of successive decline, those of gold, silver, steel, and iron, but with an important difference. Their cosmic cycle culminates in a cataclysmic fire, which destroys and purifies the world, then reborn in a new Golden Age.

Iron is frequently taboo. Frazer's *Golden Bough* cites a dozen examples: the Jews used no iron tool to build the Temple or to construct an altar; no iron may be brought into Greek sanctuaries; iron may not touch a king; animals may not be sacrificed by iron blades.

Iron ↔ Magnet. The mystery of the lodestone has captured human imagination for millennia. Unique in nature, the lodestone attracts iron across a distance, exerts a force without touching its object, and draws iron to it as if by magical sympathy. The iron seems to *want* to join the magnet. For Thales, writing in the sixth century BCE, acclaimed as the first of the Greek philosopher-scientists, the magnet possesses a soul because it moves iron—an inanimate thing endowed with soul, thus all things have souls, and things are full of gods, even a stone has motive force. Life and divinity permeate the world. Magnetism involves a secret and invisible power, like magic, a power of attraction and sympathy. A modern of the Age of Newton finds it difficult to appreciate how radical is the problem posed by the magnet: how might Nature exert a force across a distance? For in every other case, excepting a few rarities such as the vacuum and amber (static electricity), an object can influence another only by touching or striking it.

The magnet illustrates the close relation between celestial and mundane powers, the link between astrology and alchemy. Marsilio Ficino, Renaissance physician, translator of Plato and of Hermes Trismegistus, leader of the Florentine Platonic Academy under the Medici, among the greatest catalysts of Italian Humanism, writes:

We see how sailors on watch use a magnet with a needle balanced to move the Bear Star as an indication
where the Pole is, the magnet drawing them there,
because the power of the Bear Star is still in this stone.
This power is infused into it from the beginning, but
it is also continuously fed by the rays of the Bear Star.

The power of magnetic attraction and repulsion generates a metaphor that stimulated pharmacologic thinking for
centuries. Pliny the Elder (first century CE), introduces the
section of his *Natural History* devoted to drugs by expound-
ing on the metaphor:

In matters related to the fundamental principles of
things the Greeks have employed the terms "sympathy"
and "antipathy," as, for example, in the cases of water
putting out fire, the sun swallowing up water, or the
moon generating water. The sun and moon are eclipsed,
each through the transgression of the other. To turn
from heavenly things, magnetite attracts iron while
another type of stone repels it.

The Greco-Roman physician Galen also writes that
medications work by their power of attraction, like a lodestone. Attraction and repulsion, sympathy and antipathy—
here is the essence of magical thinking, also of astrological
thinking, also of alchemical thinking. It forms the basis of
Renaissance herbal pharmacy. Sympathy is the hidden relation shared among related things, the energy that connects
the manifold levels of the cosmos, and the attraction between
two elements. Sympathy, in magic, empowers the magus to
manipulate a thing by incantations of its name and empowers the voodooist to control a person by his hair clippings or
his effigy. Sympathy, in astrology, constitutes the links in the
Great Chain of Being. Sympathy, in alchemy, is the unity and

relatedness of the diverse objects of nature. The physician, viewed in this context, can treat disease by drawing on a concordance of cosmic energy between a drug and the stars.

The great compendium of Renaissance knowledge natural and supernatural, the *Magia Naturalis* of the Neapolitan Giambattista della Porta (1558), considers natural magic as the highest form in a continuum of knowledge about things, not a realm apart. Della Porta, founder of Europe's first scientific society, investigates equally natural phenomena and their quasi-supernatural correlations. His chapter on magnets proceeds from ordinary considerations, such as attraction/repulsion and polarity, to ascend through more complex observations, such as operation of magnetic force through barriers, until arriving at such extraordinary properties as the reuniting of estranged couples and the induction of melancholy.

Magnets and medicine again intersect in the person of William Gilbert, personal physician to Elizabeth I and James I, also one of the leading scientists of the era and a pioneer in the study of magnetism. His magnum opus, *On the Magnet, Magnetic Bodies, and the Great Magnet of the Earth* (1601), compiles all that was then known of magnetic attraction and the magnetic properties of the Earth itself.

And then we return to the Faustian figure of Paracelsus, a physician equally versed in practical mineralogy, speculative alchemy, Neoplatonist astrology, and clinical medicine, a man simultaneously grounded and airborne. Jung calls him a "whirlwind" and a "volcano," nicely capturing the turbulent and violent mixture of earth and air. His admirers and disciples praise him as the father, variously, of medicinal chemistry, anti-academic empiricism, and learned (rather than barbershop) surgery. His critics, and there have been many from his lifetime onwards, have impugned him as a mystic, blasphemer, bombast, lunatic egoist, iconoclast, obscurantist, and speculative troublemaker. He makes an easy screen for projecting one's fantasies—chemistry for the chemist, mysticism for the mystic, homeopathy for the homeopath. Like Faust, he sought much, reached far, and overreached. But it is precisely his weird and fateful combination of practical and magical–alchemical–astrologic knowledge that both encapsulates the intellectual paradoxes of his era and lays the groundwork for future scientific and medical discovery. He is a storm and a provocation.

Fascinated by the mine and the smithy, Paracelsus revives the Greek Hephaestus in the figure of his Roman analogue Vulcan, a god of fiery transformation, releasing pure metal from its drossy ore, releasing the remedy from its herb. "This is alchemy, and this is the office of Vulcan; he is the apothecary and chemist of the medicine."

Paracelsus was also the first European to prescribe iron as a medicine. He advocated the metal as a treatment for weakness; and iron indeed treats weakness when the ailment is caused by iron–deficiency anemia, but that is not the concept the Renaissance physician has in mind. Iron is the element of Mars, red like Mars, virile like Mars, hard, obdurate. The weak patient benefits from an infusion of the Martial spirit, for the energies of the body correspond to the energies of the cosmos. The objects of nature contain an invisible virtue, the "fifth essence" or "quintessence," that the physician discovers and applies to the treatment of disease. The goal of medical alchemy is not to transform base metal into gold, but to use the immanent correspondences among the things of nature to transform disease into health. If disease derives from corruption, then health is restored through purification. The philosopher's stone is thus the elixir of life.

For advocates and detractors alike, Paracelsus dealt a deathblow to the humoral system of scholarly medicine.

Minerals and chemicals became established treatments for diseases. By the seventeenth century, such medical luminaries as Sydenham were prescribing iron for the treatment of chlorosis, the green sickness of maidens. A few generations later, chemists found that a magnet would attract blood that had been burnt to ash—blood must contain iron and must be largely iron. The subsequent two centuries weave the separate strains together. Blood is iron, iron treats weakness, iron treats pallor, pallid weakness is blood deficiency, which is iron deficiency. Even today, the tired patient—and there are many, very many, who consult the physician because of fatigue—asks if taking iron supplements would help. Advertisements for Geritol® once offered cures for iron-poor, tired blood.

Science marches forward, vanquishing ignorance, superstition, and speculation in the progressive triumph of rational empiricism. Commerce lends its ready hand.

The mystery falls away—or does it? The patient who is ill seeks a biomechanical solution to his biomechanical problem, to be sure, but sometimes also something more, and especially in severe or mortal illness—a transmutation, a purification, a yearning, an alchemy. Not *turn me into something else*, not *turn my iron to gold*, rather *cast out this dross which is my disease, my fatality*.

If a star were to burn entirely to ash, the cinders would consist of iron. Astrochemists imagine that in some incomprehensibly distant future, perhaps 10^{100} years hence—ten thousand trillion trillion trillion trillion trillion trillion trillion trillion years from now—the elements will all decay into a common form, which should be the element iron, clouds of iron atoms. In that day (but there will be no day), iron alone will rise apart from the cosmic void, until that sturdy ruddy metal too shall fade away, and all shall again be nothing.

13. Bloodletting

THE ANCIENT PRACTICE OF BLOODLETTING IS AN ACT OF unreason. For many thousands of years, the healer has spilled the patient's blood, methodically, with therapeutic intention. One binds the upper arm, usually, and incises a large vein inside the bend of the elbow, a place beneath notice. (Here one finds one of those many body places that everyday language leaves unnamed. The technical language of medicine calls it the antecubital fossa.) The lancet is quick. The blood spills out into a basin, perhaps a few ounces, perhaps more, and then the band is released and the wound staunched. From unrecorded history to the mid-nineteenth century, medicine has repeated with little variation these same essential steps.

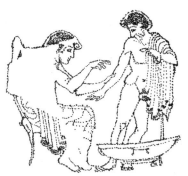

One strains to find a possible physiologic or biomechanical benefit to bloodletting. In most instances, removing a small amount of blood would have minimal biological

the tasks of the shaman is to decide if a cure requires
￼e, and if so what kind and form. Thus may the healer
￼he patient's balance of spiritual forces.
￼the same time, blood is taboo, untouchable. Blood
￼ stains. For Heraclitus, writing about 500 BCE, "They
￼purify themselves of blood-guilt by defiling them-
￼ith blood, as though one who had stepped into mud
￼ wash with mud."
￼e healer lets the patient's blood, induces anemia, saps the
￼e. "Sap," the word embodies the mystery: sap is the tree's
￼d, to sap is to draw it off and render it useful. No one
￼wever, what happens to the blood of the phlebotomized
 In most medical instances, one imagines, the blood is
￼discarded. Does this too echo the ancient ritual of spilling
￼od on the ground, blood sacrifice to Mother Earth or to
￼her infinite incarnations? The receiving vessel, in contrast,
￼notice. The surgeon-barber's symbol was his basin, useful
￼ering, useful for phlebotomy. In *Don Quixote*, the barber's
￼ecomes the golden helmet of Mambrino. In the Grail
￼, the chalice that receives the blood of the crucified Christ
￼es the goal of the quest, both the highest ideal of chival-
￼ a magical restorative of youth and everlasting life. The
￼g of Christ's side, otherwise unnecessary to his execution,
￼rms the nearly bloodless crucifixion into a blood sacrifice,
￼ted in the Eucharist.
￼ood and wine are ancient correlates. In French, blood-
￼ is *"la saignée."* The same word describes a process in
￼g rosé wine, in which a portion of red wine is drawn
￼er limited contact with the grape skins.

￼Medical theorists of whatever their era provided explana-
￼for bloodletting. For some, to remove blood was to expel
￼sease-causing demon, contagion, or principle. For others,
￼ving that in many diseases the patient is hot, to eliminate

effect, perhaps none at all. True, there are a few conditions, such as congestive heart failure or hereditary hemochromatosis, that might improve if the patient's blood volume were reduced. But for most illnesses, losing blood would prove more harmful than otherwise, as best the modern medical mind can imagine. The consequence is anemia, which weakens the patient and saps his strength.

Why, then, have healers performed this seemingly useless practice for millennia? Benighted superstition, one modern might say; ignorance, another. Or perhaps it was helpful for the doctor to do *something*, anything, rather that sit helplessly beside the patient and do nothing at all. At minimum, the patient reacts physiologically to bleeding: the pulse quickens, the color pales, something is happening. Maybe the something is good.

One must reach beyond physiology and beyond reason. Bloodletting is blood sacrifice.

If *Homo sapiens* evolved some 400,000 years ago, and agriculture began 10,000 years ago, then for perhaps ninety-seven percent of its history our species has fed itself from hunting, scavenging, and gathering. Survival required the slaying of animals, the kill. The hunter slays his prey and spills its blood.

Sacrificial ritual reenacts this central event. Amidst great ceremony, the priest slays the sacrificial victim, the ram, the goat, the bull, the ox, the sheep, the horse (in Vedic religion), the cock (especially in Greek medicine). The people have assembled in witness and participation. The animal, chosen and adorned, is led to the altar. Following the ancient ordinances of his society or religion, the priest draws his blade, flint or bronze or steel, he cuts the throat in a single motion and spills the blood, which flows into a basin or chalice or onto the bare ground. The animal is butchered, cooked (usually), and eaten. Usually all partake, sometimes only the men, sometimes only the elect.

In the new brief era of agricultural man, the communal feast provides one of the year's only occasions for eating meat. In modern America, the major holidays of Thanksgiving, Christmas, Easter (and Passover and 'Īd al-Fitr) center on a feast. Even Independence Day celebrates equally the parade and the backyard barbecue, when Dad grills burgers and hot dogs. Halloween, now the second greatest holiday of the American calendar, as measured in consumer spending, is a feast of candy, a collective gorge for children, a sugar glut.

Holocaust is a different kind of sacrificial ritual, the offering is burnt whole, burnt to nothing. The gods addressed are those of the underworld, there is no feast and no celebration.

The manner of sacrifice, the cutting of the throat, maximizes the bloodshed. There are many ways to kill a beast, but severing the vessels of the neck, the carotid arteries and the jugular veins, guarantees that much blood will flow. This remains the method prescribed for butchering by Jewish kosher law and Muslim halāl law, which require that the animal be fully bled. For these religions, *all* meat must be sanctified.

Sacrifice is sacred and dark, confronting the awful conjunction of living and dying. Might the victim be not a beast but a person? Jehovah, in what is for me the most terrifying moment in Scripture, requires Abraham to sacrifice his son Isaac, then substitutes a ram at the last instant. The Aztecs, most famously, but also the Mayans and Incans, sacrificed humans atop their altars. Other cultures have generally limited human sacrifice to those taken in war. The Roman triumph publicly paraded the vanquished, as Caesar did Vercingetorix, the leader whom he then slew.

Did the Greeks perform human sacrifice? Their myths tell how Agamemnon sacrificed his daughter Iphigenia to propitiate the offended goddess Artemis and advance the war on

Troy, how Tantalus killed his son Pel[...] banqueting gods; but the first was a [...] abomination. These were actions ou[...] als, in contrast, refer to the real poss[...] Plato alludes to a legend of human [...] Lycaean Zeus in Arcadia, and elsewh[...] ued "persistence of human sacrifice t[...] ters" without saying where those qu[...] to his own life were practices surro[...] criminal or a citizen chosen for his e[...] mity, who was feasted, led in proces[...] cast out. Some say that the *pharmakos* [...] ers that he was thrown into the sea, st[...] alive. Apollo seems so bright a go[...] Thargelia, involved the ritual murder [...]

Oedipus himself resembles a *ph[...] of Sophocles, a plague besets Thebes, [...] to be the presence of the polluted h[...] be expelled.

The word probably stems from *ph[...] poison or spell, a shadowy link of med[...] sion, and ritual. In modern Greek, *pha[...]

Sacrifice is "*sacrificium*," a Latin wo[...] making, the performance of a sacred [...] sacred, the something made sacred. The [...] deriving ultimately from fumigation, t[...] offering, the fragrant odor that drifts up [...] the appetites of gods and men. And to [...] is to consecrate with blood.

For those who believe that illness i[...] natural being, be it god, ghost, or demo[...] a benevolent deity or placate a malevo[...] fice is a gift to the gods that obliges [...]

hot blood allowed the patient to cool. For physiologists of the four humors, to withdraw the sanguinous humor conduced to health by adjusting the patient's overall constitution.

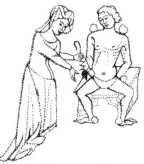

Thus Maimonides, to cite one of many possible examples, writes in the twelfth century that bloodletting aims at "clarification of the blood and rectifications of the temperament of the liver so that good blood flow is generated."

Who should bleed the patient? The earliest practitioner of the craft was the shaman. During classical antiquity, the duty fell to the physician, or often to the householder. Practical manuals of the era instructed the paterfamilias how and when to perform the task. During the European Middle Ages, the bloodletter was often a barber, whose razor and basin could serve the multiple functions of haircutting, shaving, phlebotomy, and minor surgery. When a papal decree of 1163 forbade clergy to shed blood, the surgeon-barber became a fixture of European society, lasting for hundreds of years. Only in the eighteenth century, in urbane societies, and quite later in the frontiers, did surgeons break off as a separate profession. Yet the memory of the surgeon-barber lives on in the red-and-white barbershop pole, even today the insignia of the haircutters and vestige of the bloodletters.

Leeches reverse the logic of sacrifice by performing bloodletting without bloodshed. Whatever their era, they appear modern and sanitary. In Old English, a leech was a physician, and so old was the practice of medicinal leechcraft that etymologists are uncertain whether *leech* first meant the doctor or the bloodsucking annelid. The practice reached its apogee in the early nineteenth century, when France imported as many as 42 million leeches annually (in 1833) for medicinal purposes. Leeches may be making a comeback. They work wonderfully for evacuating certain bruises. The human response ranges from revulsion (witness Bogart in *The African Queen*) to fascination: they inject a local anesthetic, to keep the host unaware of its piggyback parasite, and an anticoagulant to keep the blood flowing. Both are the subjects of current scientific investigation.

Whether performed by leeches or phlebotomy, bloodletting could be perilous, even malicious. In Calderón's tragedy *El Médico de su Honra* (*The Physician of his Honor*, 1635), a play replete with images of pallor, bleeding, and medicine, a husband who fears that his wife has dishonored him compels a surgeon to bleed her to death. George Washington probably died (1799) from the effects of excessive bloodletting. His death provided a very public demonstration of the hazards of the harsh, violent cures then called heroic medicine, and did much to stimulate the gentler reforms of the century that followed.

Come the new medical sciences of the nineteenth century, bloodletting no longer stood scrutiny. In 1828, the French physician Pierre Charles Alexandre Louis, an early champion of statistical methods in medicine, published his *Researches on the Effects of Bloodletting*, in which he argued that bloodletting has only modest effectiveness. The ancient therapy soon passed by the wayside.

Or did it?

First, if you visit a modern doctor, you will usually have a blood test. One binds your upper arm, penetrates the vein, removes a few ounces, releases the band, and staunches the wound. The action has changed little, though the blood is not spilled on the ground but rather sent to the laboratory for analysis. The chalice is wholly secular.

If you enter a hospital, the same phlebotomy happens daily, and often several times daily. Often so much blood is removed over a period of days that the patient becomes anemic and requires transfusion. (Also in Hippocratic times, a man might sometimes be bled to bloodlessness.) No matter—the phlebotomizing imperative must continue unimpeded. One might well ask if the doctors overdo their blood tests. The intern, who is usually the one responsible for ordering tests, might be chastised on rounds for ordering too few but seldom for ordering too many. How clever that he thought of some improbable or rare disease and tested for it, even if the result was normal. How diligent that he rechecked the test that was normal yesterday and the day before; how reassuring to find it normal once again.

What happens to the blood once the hospital has finished its tests? Into the autoclave, a medicinal furnace, burnt to nothingness, holocaust, ancient of days.

Second is the phenomenon of blood donation. September 11, 2001, was a brilliant clear day in New York and Washington. The attacks occurred in the morning. By noon, thousands had lined up, spontaneously and unbidden, to donate their blood. Even when it became known, over the ensuing days, that survivors were few and the demand for blood transfusion small, still the people came. Many were turned away. For the first and only time in its history, the New York Blood Center had a surplus of blood, more that it could use. Much that was donated then was ultimately discarded.

Blood donation is generally a communal act, one of the few to penetrate the shell of the modern monad-citizen. Organized by the volunteer fire department, by the labor union, by the Rotary Club, blood drives provide one of the only public occasions for organized, selfless giving. The donor has nothing to gain, besides a t-shirt and a sense of civic benevolence. But the ceremony of blood donation echoes the ancient sacrifice. The donor gives of his blood, and even partakes of a stylized feast, the comedy of cookies and apple juice that follows the diminutive ordeal. (Why a comedy? Because all the donor needs is water, and perhaps a little salt. The sugar is superfluous, a child's reward. The cookies, in an age of high cholesterol, do more harm than good.)

The bandage used to wrap the arm after blood donation is unlike those used in other medical instances, ostentatiously colored rather than white, bulky rather than trim. One could tell something about the temperament of a man by observing whether, after donating blood, he keeps his sleeve rolled up to display the bandage to passersby or instead buttons his cuffs.

Donating blood is a *self*-sacrificing act, transferred to the sphere of health and disease. It confronts the donor's anxiety about illness and blood loss, it "offers the highly tensed heart an opportunity to relieve itself through this self-denial."

Giving blood, whether the ancient's bloodletting, the modern's blood test, or the civic club's blood drive, is an offering, a gift, and a sacrifice. Inherent in all sacrifice are the notions of a gift to the gods and of the promotion of friendship among the communicants. We propitiate the violent demons of sickness and fend off their assault. So too we perform atonement, so too we expiate our own bloodguilt. The ritual spilling of blood enacts, in the words of Walter Burkert, "the two-sided nature of sacrifice—the encounter with death and the will to live," that is common to all illnesses. We who are not ill witness the sacrificial act, see the blood spilt, recall the ancient communal feast, and experience again "the pleasurable shock of survival."

14. Transfusion

A SIXTY-YEAR-OLD MAN COMES TO THE HOSPITAL BECAUSE of fever and cough. Within a few minutes, it becomes clear that he has severe pneumonia, and that the infection has spread to his bloodstream. He is admitted to the intensive care unit, where he is to spend the next three weeks battling for his life. In the course of his illness, he develops severe anemia, the consequence of innumerable blood tests and his body's inability to manufacture new red blood cells while severely ill. What is to be done?

The answer, of course, is blood transfusion. Volunteers have donated their blood, which will now be infused into the sick man. This will correct his anemia and improve both his strength, in general terms, and his ability to deliver oxygen to his embattled tissues, in specific terms.

The doctors must ask his permission to transfuse blood, and he must sign a consent form. Why, when he is so near death? Why is blood transfusion set aside as an extraordinary measure, so unlike the infusion of antibiotics that may be equally risky?

There are practical considerations, as always. Blood transfusion carries the risk of transmitting blood-borne infections. First among these is infectious hepatitis, which can lead to cirrhosis of the liver. More ominous is HIV, although modern testing has virtually eliminated this risk. Others lurk in the background: syphilis, bovine encephalitis (mad cow disease), Creutzfeld-Jakob disease, and a host of others.

Historically, efforts to transfuse blood have been fraught with peril. If blood means life and vigor, then transferring the blood of a vigorous youth into an ailing old man seems intuitively obvious. Easier said than done. Anno Domini 1492—that *annus mirabilis* that witnessed Columbus's first voyage, the unification of Spain, the expulsion of the Moors and the Jews, the births of Margaret of Navarre and of Pietro Aretino, the deaths of Lorenzo de' Medici and of Piero della Francesca—also bore sad witness to the death of Pope Innocent VIII. According to the contemporary lawyer Stefano Infessura, there was an unnamed Jewish physician who tried to revive the dying Pope, otherwise famous for fathering numerous illegitimate children, condemning Pico della Mirandola, and appointing Torquemada to head the Inquisition, by giving him the blood of three boys. It is unclear whether the blood was to be drunk or infused, but the story goes that the boys were all paid a ducat, and that all three died. So did the Pope. The physician fled. The story, reported in Infessura's *Diaries of the City of Rome*, is otherwise unverified and is strenuously contested by such authorities as the *Catholic Encyclopedia*. However, it does reflect the uncertainties and suspicions encircling the first account of blood transfusion.

It was an alchemist, not too surprisingly, who proposed the next step. The German physician Andreas Libavius authored *Alchymia* (1606), called by some the first textbook of chemistry, and also suggested invigorating an old man by infusing him with the blood of a youth. It is doubtful whether the experiment actually took place.

Christopher Wren (1632–1723) belonged to an age when a man might be expected to know many things. England's greatest architect, he also designed instruments and performed experiments for infusing liquids into the veins of animals. His fellow students at Westminster School and then Oxford included young men who were to become the philosopher John Locke, the physicist Robert Hooke, and the physician Richard Lower. Lower studied the circulation and applied Wren's techniques to transfuse blood, demonstrating the successful transfer of blood from a mastiff to an exsanguinated (smaller) dog before the Royal Society in 1665. The diarist Samuel Pepys describes a similar demonstration in his entry for November 14, 1666, which reads,

> Dr Croone told me, that at the meeting at Gresham College to-night (which it seems, they now have every Wednesday again,) there was a pretty experiment of the blood of one dog let out (till he died) into the body of another on one side, while all his own run out on the other side. The first died upon the place, and the other very well, and likely to do well. This did give occasion to many pretty wishes, as of the blood of a Quaker to be let into an Archbishop, and such like; but, as Dr Croone says, may, if it takes, be of mighty use to man's health, for the amending of bad blood by borrowing from a better body.

In 1667, Lower transfused blood from a sheep into a man, Arthur Coga, in an attempt to treat the patient's "harmless form of insanity." If the trial failed to improve the "very freakish and extravagant man," neither did it hurt him. We are not told what became of the sheep. Coga, "whose brain was a little too warm," wrote of the experience (in Latin), and Pepys described it in his diary entry for November 21, 1667. Not so salutary were the French experiments of Jean Baptiste Denis, who preceded Lower's human trial by a few months in transfusing blood from a lamb into a man. Although some recipients survived, some died, and the practice was banned.

Only in the nineteenth century did physicians try again to transfuse blood, this time from human to human, and for the entirely different purpose of resuscitating women hemorrhaging in childbirth. Some lived, some died, and by the beginning of the next century the reasons became understood: blood fell into distinct groups that could not be mixed, and successful transfusion required matching the types. The ensuing decades saw the advent of preservatives and other technical advances that made blood transfusion simple, widespread, and rather ordinary.

Indeed, doctors might order transfusions all too readily. A landmark study showed that patients in intensive care units actually did better when transfusions were limited to those with severe anemia, rather than moderate anemia.

A transfusion, if ordinary, remains fearful. Might the patient receive bad blood? If so, bad *how*? Bad because it carried a hidden infection, bad because it came from an undesirable of some sort, bad because it came from the wrong kind of person? When donors were paid for their blood donations, a practice that ended not too long ago, a disproportionate number came from poor or drug-using populations in which the rate of infectious hepatitis was high. Here, as often, infection and undesirability intersect. Different were the concerns about transfusion and race, which raised questions of contamination, eugenics, and miscegenation. The American Red Cross segregated donated blood by race for several decades and initially (1941) refused to accept blood donations from Negro donors for military use in World War II. As late as 1960, the Georgia House of Representatives passed a bill (107 to 2) that would make interracial transfusion illegal. These measures did not proceed without protest. Witness, for example, the songwriter Yip Harburg, lyricist of "Somewhere Over the Rainbow" and "Brother, Can You Spare a Dime," who lampooned transfusion segregation in his "Free and Equal Blues," set to the tune of the old "St. James Infirmary Blues" and popularized by the singer Josh White.

★   ★   ★

Appropriating the blood of another creature has long been thought to vivify the recipient. In *The Odyssey*, the ghost of Tiresias will speak to Odysseus only after drinking the blood of a sacrificed ram. The vampire of legend, of course, can live only by drinking human blood. Stranger still is the case of Elizabeth Bathory (1560–1614), a Hungarian countess who tortured and murdered young women and who, in later folklore, sought to rejuvenate herself by bathing in her victims' blood. Such tales recognize the vital power of blood but also cast a ghoulish aura about its transfer from one person to another.

The strange mixing of body elements has captured the imagination for centuries. The story is told of Saints Cosmas and Damian, the patron saints of medicine in the Catholic tradition, how they miraculously removed the diseased leg of a (white) man and replaced it with the otherwise healthy leg of a recently deceased Ethiopian. More specifically, this was the dream vision of a devout believer in the Church of Sts. Cosmas and Damian in Rome, who then awoke to find that a hale black leg had replaced his sick white leg. Fra Angelico painted the scene, replacing the otherwise anonymous patient with the emperor Justinian, and so did other Renaissance painters. The scene harkens back to the ancient Greek tradition of temple healing, a dream vision of miraculous cure mediated by the healing god. Similarly, in a second legend of the miraculous healing of Cosmas and Damian, a serpent entered the mouth of a farmer asleep in a field. That evening, "when the pain and anguish increased he went to the church of the saints, and fell suddenly asleep, and then the serpent issued out of his mouth like as it had entered."

Even today, people facing transfusion often request that the donor be a friend or family member, even though receiving such blood does not reduce the risk of infection. Your neighbor, after all, might have hepatitis C as well as the next man. But the blood of a known donor feels less strange. Or: a patient planning for elective surgery might donate his own blood, to be replaced if needed during the operation. No strangeness here at all.

The steps in actually administering a blood transfusion add to its emotional charge and sanctity. The doctor must discuss with the patient the risks, benefits, and alternatives to transfusion. The patient must sign a consent form, not merely accede. To infuse the blood, two nurses must be present, one to read the identification information on the bag itself, one to confirm the patient's identity. Again the ritualized actions create a ceremony, this time dedicated to therapy rather than diagnosis.

Blood transfusion is beset with worry, partly the result of rational concerns, partly of deep fears. These remember the early blood transfusions, real or imagined, which were not treatments for anemia, of course, or even for pallor, but rather for infirmity, especially the debility of old age, and for weakmindedness. The premise was that youthful, healthy blood contained some vital principle that could invigorate the frail and revitalize the moribund. If I need blood my own blood is bad, I am infirm, debilitated, devitalized, toxified. But if I receive blood so might the infusion be bad blood, infected, contaminated, rendered somehow evil, and so might I be rendered somehow wrong, somehow other, somehow not myself, strange, estranged, another creature's lifeblood circulating within me.

15. Is Anemia Good for You?

ANEMIA, CONCEIVED AS A DEFICIENCY OF BLOOD, IS DEFINED as a numerical deviation. Whoever has a hemoglobin measurement below a certain cutoff has anemia. In men, the lower cutoff is 14 g/dL (grams per deciliter). Anemia is bad, anemia is a disease, or more precisely a sign of disease (which amounts to the same thing). Doctors therefore care about anemia, they are alarmed when it appears, they search for the disease that caused it.

The body, in contrast, doesn't care about anemia, not exactly. What the body cares about is oxygen delivery to tissues. Oxygen delivery depends on the hemoglobin count, in part, but also on how well blood flows from the heart, through the arteries and capillaries, to the cells. And this latter property, how well the blood flows, depends on its viscosity.

Viscosity actually *improves* in anemia. To have fewer red blood cells means that the blood is less densely packed and passes more easily through the vessels. There is a trade-off. A higher blood count means greater oxygen-carrying capacity but less flow, while a lower blood count means lower oxygen-carrying capacity but more flow. Somewhere in between, there must be a happy medium.

And so there is. Oxygen delivery to tissues is optimal when the hemoglobin count is about 10 g/dL. That must be the healthiest level, no?

No, says Medicine, the healthy level is a hemoglobin count greater than 14 g/dL, below that level is disease. Strange and stranger, might it be better to have the disease, than not?

The New York Times, November 16, 2006: "Heart Risk Seen in Drug for Anemia." This article, prominently featured on the front page of the Business Day section, reported on two studies being published that day in *The New England Journal of Medicine*. The reports, evidently deemed especially pertinent to the newspaper's financial readership, found that a group of drugs used to raise the blood count in patients with mild or moderate anemia not only provides no benefit but could actually increase the risk of heart attack and death. The lead author of the second study, reported the *Times*, "said that the results were surprising."

Not so surprising, seen from a different perspective. One might well have predicted that a higher blood count could increase the viscosity of blood, reduce its flow, increase the propensity of blood to clot, and cause the vascular occlusions of heart attack and stroke.

And there is an added twist: it appears, not altogether surprisingly, that doctors order these medicines in higher doses in large, for-profit dialysis chain facilities than in non-profit dialysis clinics. Apparently financial interest, not only clinical interest, plays a role in the decision.

Read at face value, the story is a cautionary tale about how the treatment of a medical condition might make matters worse, rather than better. Reading its subtexts, one might puzzle over several ramifications.

First, conflict arises between two concepts of normal, the statistical and the teleological. A statistical, normative definition states that health and disease consist in numerical values. Those that fall within a standard distribution are normal and healthy, while those that fall outside the distribution are abnormal and diseased. A teleological definition states that health and disease consist in whatever benefits the organism. Health resides in whatever is advantageous and good, while disease resides in whatever is disadvantageous and bad. In the case of anemia, a hemoglobin value of 11 g/dL, for example, constitutes disease by the statistical definition but health by the teleological definition.

Statistical and teleological considerations can easily leak over into a third realm, constituted by moral definitions of normal and abnormal, which should have little place in considering health and disease. "Your blood count is good" is a dangerous statement that constructs a dangerous moral paradigm.

Doctors, naturally, find it easier to decide which numbers are statistically abnormal than what is good and bad for a patient. Indeed, modern times would consider the physician who spoke of what is good and bad for the patient as woefully paternalistic, a serious no-no.

Second, the "normal" range is defined from statistical samples in the here and now, using "here" as the industrial worlds of Europe, North America, and the Pacific Rim, and "now" as the last hundred years or so. People in other places and in earlier times have generally had lower blood counts. Perhaps they were sick, the victims of iron deficiency, parasitic worms, chronic infections, and the like.

Or perhaps they were well, and their lower hemoglobin values were *healthier* than our higher numbers. What most threatens the health of a modern is not hemorrhage, not attack by a saber-toothed tiger, but rather thrombosis, the occlusion of an artery, the essential event in heart attack and stroke. Are our higher hemoglobin values thus a form of hematological obesity, a *too-muchness* in the blood, too much iron (too much meat), or even too few parasites? Our vascular systems evolved to work better under different conditions, when our hemoglobin counts were lower.

Third, the modern definitions of anemia may represent a kind of medical colonialism, an instance of the "advanced" countries dictating values to the "primitives." Just as a "third world" reduced diet decreases the risk of heart attack and stroke, so might a reduced hemoglobin decrease risk. In diet, as in anemia, there should be a middle ground between deficiency and glut.

Fourth, similarly, many older patients develop mild anemia. The doctor conceives this as a signal of disease, but perhaps instead it is an adaptive measure to help prevent heart attack and stroke.

Fifth, bleeding the patient—might this antique practice make sense after all? The surgeon-barber who bled his patient induced anemia, thinned the blood, and probably, if unwittingly, reduced the chance of heart attack and stroke. It seems our eager ridicule must once again take pause.

Might donating blood benefit the donor, beyond altruistic motives? Some studies have shown just that, finding lower rates of heart disease in persons who donate blood regularly. One additional explanation for this observation is that iron increases the body's production of free radicals, which can attack healthy cells, so that reducing iron might reduce cellular damage.

Sixth, if a doctor tells you something bad, think twice: bad number or bad health? Bad for him, the doctor, or bad for *me*?

Doctors, viewing another person the patient, viewing another place the otherworld, viewing another time the past, viewing another lifetime the aged, find themselves in a quandary, poised between a sense of what *is* and what *ought* to be. Reflection and humility, again and again, are the proper companions of *ought*.

16. The Blood of the Medusa

MEDUSA THE GORGON HAD BEEN A BEAUTIFUL MAIDEN. Medusa the Gorgon became a winged monster, terrible and fearful, with round face, tusk-like fangs, protruding tongue, and snakes for hair. Perseus the hero cut off her head. From the severed neck spouted two streams of blood, carefully collected by the goddess Athena. One vial healed, the other killed.

Heroes slay monsters. It is the business of heroes to kill monsters, the slaying of monsters ranks among the hero's defining acts. Theseus kills the Minotaur, Heracles kills Geryon, Bellerophon kills the Chimera, Oedipus kills the Sphinx, Beowulf kills Grendel, St. Martha kills La Tarasque. Often the nemesis is a dragon, as for Cadmus, Daniel (in the apocryphal *Bel and the Dragon*), Siegfried (the Norse Sigurd), St. Michael, St. George, King Arthur, and Tristan. And often the monster is a great serpent, whether of land or sea, sometimes blending into the dragon motif. Gilgamesh, in the oldest Sumerian version, slays the giant serpent Kur coiled about the base of the world tree. Marduk, chief god of the Babylonians, kills the sea snake Tiamat and splits her in two, one part becoming heaven and the other earth. Each night the Egyptian Seth kills the underworld serpent Apopis, who reappears the next night again to do battle. The Canaanite Baal slays the sea serpent Yamm, Jehovah slays Leviathan, Apollo slays the serpent Python who guards the Oracle at Delphi, thus making it his own. Heracles, again, kills Hydra. Thor kills Jormungard, Midgardsorm, the Midgard serpent, who drowns the thunder god in venom, the twilight of the gods.

The hero is male, the monster belongs to either sex, the weapon is a sword, club, spear, lance, arrow.

And Perseus, hero, eponymous founder of the Persians, kills the Gorgon Medusa, whose hair was hissing snakes.

Danaë the maiden was kept in a bronze room, a prison, the king her father put her there, an oracle had prophesied that his grandson would overthrow him. Zeus visited her in a golden beam of light, she conceived, the king cast the infant boy and mother to sea in a wooden chest. They drifted to an island, they lived, a fisherman received them, the son was Perseus the hero.

The island's king, wooing Danaë and fearing her son, sets Perseus an impossible task, to bring back the head of Medusa. Once a beautiful maid, Medusa had lain with the sea god Poseidon in the temple of Athena, desecrating the sanctuary, and the outraged goddess turned the girl's hair to snakes. Her gaze turns mortals to stone. With divine assistance, carried by winged boots, Perseus slays the Gorgon, he cuts off her head.

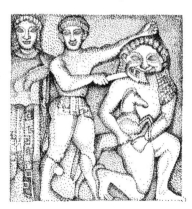

Fleeing Medusa's two immortal Gorgon sisters, Perseus goes on to free the princess Andromeda, who is to be sacrificed to a sea monster. He marries her, he turns her impious parents to stone. They look down upon us evermore, the constellations Cepheus the father, Cassiopeia the mother, Andromeda the sacrificial bride, Cetus the monster, Pegasus the great square of the winter sky. There too stands Perseus the hero holding the Gorgon's severed head, its brightest star is Algol, an eclipsing variable that dims every three days, its name in Arabic means "head of the demon."

For the Babylonians, the constellations we know as Perseus and Cetus were Marduk and Tiamat, the story is very old, and so are the stars.

From the severed head of Medusa spring two offspring of Poseidon, the beautiful Pegasus, the monstrous Chrysaor. Pegasus was the winged horse that Bellerophon rode to kill the monster Chimera. Where his hoof struck Mt. Helicon in Boetia, there gushed forth the spring of the Hippocene, the font of poetic inspiration from which the Muses were to drink. Chrysaor became the father of Geryon, the three-headed giant whom Heracles slew, and of Echidna, the half-woman half-snake who bore a host of monsters. One such was the Chimera.

His triumphs completed, Perseus gives the Gorgon's head to Athena, who affixes the image to her shield. Others mimic the goddess. Agamemnon's shield also bears a Gorgon's head, which becomes the emblem most frequently depicted on shields in Greek vase paintings. Hector in battle terrifies his opponents with Gorgon's eyes; whether these belong to his shield or to his own visage is ambiguous.

For classical Greece, Medusa's head is a grotesque mask, a leering grinning face with tusks, tongue protruding, snakes for hair. The image rings their temples, apotropaic, warding off evil. The very earliest example of Greek pedimental sculpture, from the Temple of Artemis at Corfu, circa 570 BCE, centers on the figure of Medusa. Also in Athens, on the south wall of the Acropolis, a gilded head of Medusa the Gorgon faced and overlooked the theater. In Euripides' *Ion*, the women of the

Chorus encircle a temple and look in wonder at the figure of Athena wielding her Gorgon shield.

Medusa may also take the form of an antefix, a terracotta end plate of a roof beam.

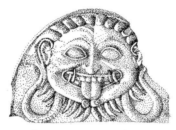

Such antefixes circle many an archaic temple, a hideous emblem on the sacred monument. They kept the roof beams from rotting.

The myth continues yet a bit further. Athena gives the two vials of blood to Asklepios, the hero-god of medicine. Or to Erichthonius, the first king of her city Athens. *One vial heals, the other kills.* The physician, whose emblem is a snake entwining a staff, goes too far. He raises the dead, he oversteps, he commits blasphemy, and Zeus strikes him dead with a thunderbolt.

In Goethe's *Faust*, the image of Medusa is the girl once loved, pale, irrecoverable, fatal, petrifying, a specter, an illusion. Shall we compare her to Health as envisioned by one who has fallen sick?

The word "medusa" comes from the Greek *medein*, to rule. Its Indo-European root is *med-*, "to take appropriate measures." Descended from the same root are the Latin *medicus*, and hence the English "medicine."

The blood of Medusa: one stream kills, the other heals. Monsters and slayers of monsters, ogres and heroes, giants and giganticides. Two offspring of Poseidon by Medusa, one bears a monster, one bears the hero who kills a monster. Always in mythologic memory the airborne hero aloft on wings, Perseus,

Bellerophon, Wotan, Hermes the god, a thousand others, an upward movement against the ponderous downward drag of thwarted desire and mortal necessity. The physician wields two vials, one kills, the other heals, killing and healing, two ends of a spectrum or a circle. Asklepios heals too far and is destroyed. Snake again, the ouroboros, the serpent that bites its tail, a circle, and which shall kill and which shall heal?

How does the hideous mask of Medusa ward off evil? How does the physician fend off evil? The Gorgon combines beauty and horror, conceived in holy and unholy love, the union of mortal and immortal. Zeus beds with Danaë in a bronze prison, the father would forbid it, love conquers all. One senses some combination of tenderness and rapture rather than rape. Poseidon beds with Medusa in a temple, outraging the gray-eyed goddess, who transforms the girl into a fiend. The god goes blameless. The doctor wears a kindly face—what then is his hideous mask, his apotropaic visage, to keep evil away?

His dwelling, the hospital, is a temple. The hospital is a place of sanctified cures, sun-filled, well aired, clean; also of suffering and death, therefore taboo, nefas, a pesthouse, a dungeon, a torture chamber, a penal colony, a leprosarium, a mortuary. The hospital is a palace and a labyrinth, a Knossus, and the physician inside is both Theseus and Minotaur.

For diseases of the blood, the specter is chemotherapy. The hematologist-oncologist is he who gives chemotherapy, and chemotherapy defines the subspecialty. This unity of the blood specialist and the cancer specialist stems not from clinical necessity but rather from a quirk in recent medical history. Cancer had always been a surgical disease, curable, if at all, by the surgeon. If extirpation was impossible, the case was fatal. However, in the 1950s, blood specialists began to treat blood diseases—above all, leukemia—with a new kind of medication, called chemotherapy. The medicines were highly toxic and derived, originally, from chemical weapons, such as nitrogen mustard gas, developed in the First World War. This was the gas that killed my soldier grandfather, and this gave the medicine that treated his son, my uncle. The term *chemotherapy* meant to contrast with surgical therapy but also bore nasty after-echoes: chemical, poison, war.

In principle, one could call any drug a form of chemotherapy, and some purists do, but most use the term to refer to cancer chemotherapy, drugs used to treat cancer. The hematologists became adept at giving medications to treat leukemia. The next step was to use medications to treat other cancers, and the hematologists administered these too. Before long, the hematologist was an oncologist, a specialist in the medical (i.e., nonsurgical) treatment of cancer. Should lung cancer be treated by a lung specialist or a cancer specialist? The answer became the latter, for he best knew the medicines that destroy the cancerous cells, and best handled their toxicities.

Conventional cancer chemotherapy is indeed poisonous. Borrowing a theme from antibiotics, its purpose is to kill. Yet unlike penicillin, which harms bacteria but not human cells, the original cancer chemotherapy drugs were harmful to *all* cells—by intent, more to cancer cells than to healthy cells. The result was drastic and had dramatic side effects: nausea, vomiting, diarrhea, hair loss, as well as the subtler anemia and susceptibility to severe infection. Many patients find the threat of side effects from chemotherapy more fearful than the cancer itself.

How is the patient to bear the monstrous side effects? Does undergoing the ordeal keep at bay the greater evil, which is the fatal disease? Does wielding the Gorgon-headed shield somehow defy and scorn the enemy? Is it a talisman, a protective evil eye?

Drugs have always carried a double sense of benevolence and malevolence. Reaching back to the most ancient roots of Indian medicine, the Vedic tradition considered an herb—like many other divine powers—to be indifferent as to whether it helped or harmed a patient. To gain the drug's goodwill, the physician-magician must supplicate and propitiate the plant through ritual and magic. Medea, half a love-struck girl, half a sorceress, keeps a box that holds both healing and deadly drugs. Indeed, the Greeks used a single word, *pharmakon*, to mean both medicine (whence our "pharmacology") and evil potion. Circe, another witchy lass, turns the men of Odysseus into beasts by giving them a "*pharmakon*." Euripides' Hermione accuses Andromache of rendering her barren with a *pharmakon*.

Also in the Persian-Arabic tradition of the Middle Ages, Ibn Sīnā (Avicenna) writes that there are four degrees of medications. The first are those whose effects are generally not appreciated, except when taken often or in large amounts. The second are more powerful but still do not disturb normal function except when taken often or in large amounts, and then only indirectly. The third directly impair normal body function but not so much as to cause damage or death. The fourth do cause damage or death. Thus, medicines for Ibn Sīnā exist along a spectrum from imperceptible to deadly. The issue here is not helpful versus harmful, rather that the increasing degrees of efficacy each heighten toxicity.

Physicians, too, tread a narrow line between help and harm. Nowhere is this more evident than in administering chemotherapy, which may well kill the patient. The Hippocratic physicians, ever mindful of clinical paradox, swore not to harm the patient, and we still swear their Oath today. Whether we uphold the Oath in insisting on aggressive "chemo"—here defanged with an affectionate nickname—to an aged and frail cancer patient can be debated. The question often forms a point of contention between the oncologist and the gentler family physician. Here too gender roles underlie the exchange: aggressive chemo is active and virile, yang, while restraint is passive and effeminate, yin. As the two physicians debate the patient's therapeutic fate, which is the more heroic?

Asklepios the hero-god used the Gorgon's blood to heal, also to revive the dead: Capaneus, Hippolytus, Tyndareus, Lycurgus, and others. For these crimes against nature and piety, Zeus destroyed him with a thunderbolt. For in that time, even the immortals, the deathless, could meet a violent end.

The physician sees what must not be seen, *don't look, don't look*, he confronts the monster whose gaze is fatal, he severs the fatal head and its fatal eyes. Upstart Nietzsche, borne on winged sandals: "We behold all things through the human head and cannot cut off this head; while the question nonetheless remains what of the world would still be there if one had cut it off?"

Medusa, a great power, beautiful and horrific, embodies heroism, embodies horror, bearing a force that heals and destroys, defiant, apotropaic, gallant, and dreadful, a glaring stone mask. Medusa, a beauty, perhaps it is her beauty and not her hideous visage that petrifies the beholder; these were the testimonies of Lucian, of Pausanias, and of Christine de Pizan. Medusa, an ancient goddess, an earth goddess, the new Olympians who replaced her in the devotions of men transformed her into a fiend. Medusa, a poem, a painting that Shelley saw in the Uffizi, "the tempestuous loveliness of terror." The face changes others to stone, the face has itself been changed to stone, impassive as the mighty goddess who wields it, she speaks to mortals, she fights beside them, she intercedes on their behalf, she chooses whom and when and where. Odysseus senses something, the goddess is speaking to him and to him alone, the others see and hear her not, he heeds her, he yields, he triumphs, the slaughter is magnificent.

V. MYTHOS / STORY

Chorus: To what kinder place than this could we come,
Suppliants bearing wool-draped branches in our hands?

—AESCHYLUS, *The Suppliant Women*

17. The Birth
of Clinical Tragedy

IN ILLNESS, THE FREE MAN BECOMES UNFREE. ONCE ABLE TO choose his own way and to determine his own path, he now labors under the rule of forces more powerful than his own. Entering the realm of sickness, a man becomes aware, and painfully, of his tenuous balance between freedom and necessity, independence and contingency, choice and fate.

Tragic drama of the fifth century BCE marks this same precarious point of balance. Its literary predecessor consisted of chorus only, originally a sacred dance, later a group of citizens reciting lyric odes in civic and religious celebration, a gesture of unison and unanimity. It was Thespis the poet, some say, who added an actor—a protagonist, a hero—standing in contradistinction to the group. Aeschylus added a second actor, and then came more. Their iambic meter sounded more proselike than the choral songs, which by contrast assumed an archaic tone. The tragic hero—Agamemnon, Orestes, Oedipus, Antigone, Pentheus—takes action but then discovers, only later, that one's decisions may have fatal consequences, and that one's own will may countenance an external compulsion, the will of the gods.

Tragedy thus creates a set of counterpoised prerogatives: the individual and the community, choice and necessity, freedom and compulsion, present and past, knowing and discovering.

* * *

At the very same time, on the island of Cos near Asia Minor, a physician named Hippocrates rose to prominence, becoming the foremost practitioner of the Hellenic world. The books that bear his name place a special emphasis on the close and personal observation of sick people, observations that are then discovered to fit into a pattern. The illness of every sick man is his own and takes its individualistic form, but the illnesses of the many may be similar to each other, and these similarities can be grouped together under the name disease. Disease is an abstraction that yet matches, with greater and lesser fidelity, the concrete suffering of an individual person. The unique contours of one's own illness thus confront the uniformity of the disease.

Epidemic, a major focus of the Hippocratic texts, writes this theme most clearly, when the entire community is threatened by the same sickness. If illness is an individual catastrophe, epidemic draws the whole community into its fold. Indeed, epidemic loomed large in the Greek mind. *The Iliad* begins in pestilence, visited on the Greek armies by Apollo, the god whose domains include music and light and *healing*. The wrath of Achilles that powers *The Iliad* stems from the undoing of this god-sent disease, an awful tangling of darkness and illumination. So too *The Oresteia* opens with the Chorus's recollection of recent plague. Complexity upon complexity: it is Apollo who orders Orestes to kill, and Apollo who pleads the hero's case before the tribunal in Athens, who sends disease, who heals.

The Suppliant Women of Aeschylus takes place in a land where pestilence and serpents once had reigned, cleansed by Apis the seer and physician, a son of Apollo.

Athens, not the city of the imagination but the place where craftsmen and tradesmen and their families lived and died, suffered a horrific plague in 430 BCE. Sophocles' *Oedipus Tyrannus*, appearing a year or so later, starts in a city beset by plague.

The trope carries forward to Rome. The penultimate tale of Ovid's *Metamorphoses* tells how the medicine god, Latinized into Aesculapius, transforms himself into a serpent and saves the city from pestilence.

Outraged Achilles, the immobilized bloodthirsty armies, the one and the many. Titanic Prometheus, shivering humankind. Apollo who sends disease and yet may bear it away. Calm Dionysius whose frenzied bacchants tear blaspheming Pentheus limb from limb. Gray-eyed Athena whose shield bears the image of a maid once beautiful whose hairs are snakes. Serpents lick clean the ears of the seer, serpents whisper cures in the temple of Asklepios, serpents slay prescient Laocoön and his hapless sons, serpents spring from the spilt blood of Medusa, a serpent (or two) enwraps a staff and forms the caduceus.

The actor, the chorus. Fear, and triumph, submission, defiance, and fear again, and awe.

As I reread these lines once more, a man has just died. I cared for him for some fifteen years, side by side through heart surgery, cancer, and the end. His family was with him when he died, suddenly, and so was I, and then I closed his lids, hoping to have proved a worthy companion. He lived well and faced his illness calmly. The Furies circled his bed, wingless Medusas twined with snakes, they grimaced hideously, and I the physician tried to fend them off, for a while, knowing that he would soon succumb, knowing too that I will someday succumb, parting from those we love. A bond between us, a titanium rod, has been broken, and has not been broken, ever.

Walt Whitman, who nursed the sick at the very same hospital where I work now, went on to tend the wounded soldiers on the Virginia battlefields of the Civil War. He wrote of many things, of men ill and dying, of men dead. He wrote "That the hands of the sisters Death and Night incessantly softly wash again, and ever again, this soil'd world," and then he writes, "a man divine as myself is dead." He wrote of comrades, and of companions, and of friends dearly loved.

Let us say that sympathy is not a kindly disposition but a radical biological event in which two separate and autonomous people feel themselves joined. In drama, this junction is the basis of catharsis. In medicine, let us call it a form of love. Our human sorrow is not that death equals annihilation, rather that we must someday part from all those whom we love.

Disease forces the hero under compulsion, from which he strives to wrest himself, attaining happy conclusion or ill, pursued by Furies that do or do not transform into Eumenides. In disease, the self-determining impulse of an individual man must confront the forces that shape or master his destiny. This is the tragic moment, and this the birth of clinical tragedy.

The bond and sympathy between the hero and the chorus are the same that join the hero and the spectator, that join the hero and the drama's author, that join the patient and the physician. The patient is the hero, necessity draws him downward, we watch and feel it, knowing little, feel it.

18. Why Again Greeks?

ONE RETURNS AGAIN AND AGAIN TO THIS ANCIENT PEOPLE of the Aegean and its rim. Why these, and not the equally worthy people of Sumeria, the Levant, India, China, or anywhere else?

First, and most obviously, the Greeks constitute our (my) visible origins. Whoever came earlier is lost in fragmented obscurity, lost. The Greeks are thus not everyone's father, but they are our father, my father, to the extent that we can know him.

Second are their infinitely rich and interwoven stories: Homer, Hesiod, Aeschylus, Sophocles, Euripides, Plato. Most likely the *Ramayana* and the *Mahabharata* are equally rich, but their stories are not my own, and Rama will not be my Odysseus, nor Arjuna my Apollo.

Third are their gods, immortal but not unflawed, deities beside whom a man can stand without falling prostrate.

Fourth is the *kouros*.

Fifth, but properly first, is the lovely book of my childhood, *D'Aulaire's Book of Greek Myths*, which I read and reread, the gods spoke, they wed mortals, they stood beside the hero and spoke to him, visible and invisible, the voice of Athena, the voice of the plank in the bow of the Argo, the presence of Zeus before Danaë, infinite riches in a little room, a sacred space on Mulberry Lane, until these gods and heroes too shall fall away.

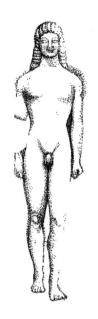

Postscript

Nay, compassion it self comes
to no great degree, if we have not felt
in some proportion, in our selves,
that which we lament and condole
in another

distortions on Donne, Meditation XXIII

Metusque, relabi

Acknowledgments

THIS BOOK WAS CONCEIVED BY ERIKA GOLDMAN, EDITORIAL DIREC-
tor of the newly spawned Bellevue Literary Press, who spoke with
me in the summer of 2006 and proposed that I write the first of her
pathographies. A pathography, in her conception, is the complete
biography of a disease, comprising its cultural, literary, mythological,
historical, and biological dimensions. The idea of a pathography
rejects the division of subject and object, of sensibility and biology,
and joins them into a whole that embraces simultaneously the subjective and objective experience of health and illness. Erika has been
a constant stimulus and support, an author's physician and surgeon
both. To Erika, then: heartfelt gratitude, tribute, and praise.

Others who have offered stimulation, goads, kicks, and con-
traries: Michael Diamond and our lifetime of conversation; Tom
Sleigh and his wonderful mind and ear; Susan Stewart and her
nuanced read of everything there is; D.W. Robertson, Jr., and John
Fleming, who taught that poems should be understood in their
historic and social contexts; Eric Cassell and Jerry Colliver, who
urge a multidimensionality in medicine; Giovanni de Simone and
his ever dialogue of life and mind. Jerome Lowenstein, the pub-
lisher of BLP; Trisha Brown, the choreographer and dancer; Burt
Barr, the video artist; Zarela Martínez, the great chef, restaurateur
and champion of Mexican culture; Anne Mendelson, the writer
and editor; and Kostas Kouris, psychologist and composer, have
also lent their support, encouragement, and helpful suggestions.

Althea Scott, for many years, and Cassia Charles, newly, have
steered my clinical practice and kept my head on straight.

My father, Charles Robert Bardes, instilled a love of the poetic
line and of rhetoric in the best sense of the word; my mother, Judith
Leopold Bardes, a love of the Greeks and their incomparable myths.
Emma Bardes, my daughter, pointed the way to the green sickness
in *Romeo and Juliet*, though I thought I knew better, to the magnan-
imous strength of melancholy, and to courage; John Bardes, my son,
to building in stone and the heartful questioning of everything.

To Barbara Kilpatrick, my wife and lifelong friend, truest
artist, all honor and thanks, love, word, and silence.

Notes and References

The translations, except where otherwise indicated, are my own.

EPIGRAPHS

5   *Distortions on Donne.* In 1627, the poet John Donne fell gravely ill. Then age fifty-four, a priest and Dean of St. Paul's Church in London, he struggled near death for several weeks. It was during and immediately after this period that he wrote his *Devotions Upon Emergent Occasions*, a set of twenty-three essays that narrate his illness and recovery. In the *distortions on Donne,* I have seized or usurped passages from the prose *Devotions* and rendered them in verse, hoping to engage what Donne's friend and biographer Isaak Walton called "the perplexities of his generous mind."

5   *Donne*, Devotions Upon Emergent Occasions. In *The Complete Poetry and Selected Prose of John Donne*, Charles M. Coffin, ed. (1952; reprint New York: Modern Library, 1994).

6   *Piers Plowman.* John Langland (attrib.). *The Vision of Piers Plowman*, Passus VI, line 102.

PROPYLAEUM

9   *Disease.* In its modern construction, *disease* refers to disordered biomechanics, while *illness* is the subjective experience of feeling unwell. While the difference is in many ways intuitive, the first to articulate the contrast was Alvan Feinstein, who identifies three different type of clinical data: *disease*, described in scientific and impersonal terms; *the host*, referring to characteristics of the patient, and *illiness*, the interaction between the disease and the host. The first to probe the concept of illness and disease as two poles in the sickness phenomenon is Eric Cassell, who has devoted his career to studying and improving he doctor-patient relationship. The concept is explored further by Arthur Kleinman.

See: Alvan R. Feinstein, MD, *Clinical Judgment* (Baltimore; Williams & Wilkins, 1967) 24–5. Eric J. Cassell, MD, *The Healer's Art: A New Approach to the Doctor-Patient Relationsip* (Philadelphia and New York: Lippincott, 1976), Arthur Kleinman, *Patients and Healers in the Context of Culture: An Exploration of the Borderland between Anthropology, Medicine, and Psychiatry* (Berkeley: University of California Press, 1980).

Neither term comprehends a word like "anemia," which neither specifies a pathophysiology nor indicates what the patient is feeling.

PREFACE

10   *Blood smear.* Drawing after a photomicrograph kindly provided by Dominick Falcone, PhD.

12   *Alieniloquium.* Alien-speak, other-speak, strange-speak. For Isidore of Seville, the great medieval encyclopedist, figural speech is to say one thing and mean another. *Etymologies* I.37.21–2; cited in D.W. Robertson, Jr., *A Preface to Chaucer: Studies in Medieval Perspectives* (Princeton: Princeton University Press, 1962), 288. For Varro, on the other hand, "alieniloquium" is "the talk of crazy persons"; cited in the 1879 *Latin Dictionary* of Charleton T. Lewis and Charles Short, *The Perseus Project,* http://www.perseus.tufts.edu. In the *Oxford English Dictionary, alieniloquy* is "a talking wide from the purpose, or not to the matter in hand."

1: DISEASIFICATION

15   *Seventy-four-year-old man.* An earlier version appeared in *Agni* 63 (2006):239–240.

17   *Popeye.* Spinach has not always been regarded as healthful. Its reputation as a uniquely valuable source of iron appears to have stemmed from an error in an 1890 German scientific paper, in which a misplaced decimal point caused the author to overestimate the vegetable's iron content by a factor of ten. Hamblin, T.J., "Fake!," *British Medical Journal* 283 (1981):1671–4. Hunter, R., "Why Popeye Took Spinach," *Lancet* 7702 (1971):746–7.

2: PALLOR

19   *Wan.* "Wann" in Old English is "dark, gloomy, black." The word then morphed into the sickly appearance of infected wounds, then sickly appearance in general, then pale—a complete turnaround. The curious history of the word, which always kept its gloomy undertones, is traced in the *Oxford English Dictionary.* "Wanhope," in Middle English, is despair.

19   *Oversensitive.* To cite an example from Poe, nearly at random: "I thought, too, that I perceived the traces of sorrow in her countenance, which was excessively, although to my taste, not unpleasingly, pale." "Dr Tarr and Prof Feather." In *The Complete Tales and Poems of Edgar Allan Poe* (New York: Modern Library, 1938).

19   *Suntan.* The fashion has prevailed ever since. "dress." Encyclopædia Britannica. *Encyclopædia Britannica 2007 Ultimate Reference Suite* (Chicago: Encyclopædia Britannica, 2007).

One wonders if the turning point was World War I, that catastrophe that darkened Europe forever. A German woman writes of her early childhood, "And when my father had to become a soldier in 1916, when he said good-bye to my mother at the train station, he reminded her never to forget to put my lace bonnet on to protect me from the sun. So that I would have a lily-white neck and a lily-white face; that was the fashion of the times for girls from good homes." So recalls the anonymous author of the 1945 diary *A Woman in Berlin: Eight Weeks in the Conquered City*. Trans. Philip Boehm (New York: Henry Holt and Company, 2005), 75.

19   *Effeminacy*. "'Sir Clerk of Oxenford,' oure Hoste sayde, / 'Ye ryde as coy and still as dooth a mayde.'" *The Canterbury Tales*, "The Clerk's Prologue," lines 1–2.

19   *Bartleby*. Herman Melville, "Bartleby, the Scrivener: A Story of Wall Street."

19   *Hazlitt*. He is so described by Edward Dowden, *The Life of Percy Bysshe Shelley* (London: Kegan Paul, Trench & Co., 1887), 100. The biographer may have unwittingly borrowed the phrase "worn and wan" from his subject's 1818 poem "Lines Written Among the Euganean Hills," line 3.

19   *Kafka. The Trial*, Chapter 1 (1914-15; published posthumously 1925). "*Diese so uncharakteristischen, blutarmen, jungen Leute.*"

20   *Why so pale and wan?* Thus begins a lyric from the fourth act of Sir John Suckling's extravagant drama *Aglaura*, first performed in 1637.

20   *Chaucer. Troilus and Criseyde*, II.551 (1374.)

20   *Greene. Pandosto, or The Triumph of Time* (1588) in *An Anthology of Elizabethan Prose Fiction*. Ed. Paul Salzman (New York: Oxford University Press, 1998), 186.

20   *Nor does Galen think highly of such men. Mixtures* II.631 in *Galen: Selected Works*. Ed. and trans. P.N. Singer (Oxford: Oxford University Press, 1997).

20   *Hamlet* Act III, scene i.

20   *Louis H. Sullivan. The Autobiography of an Idea* (New York: Dover Publications, Inc, Reprint Edition, 1956), 325.

20   *Menelaus confronts Paris. The Iliad,* Book 3, lines 33–37. The word translated as pallor is *ōchros*, signifying "pale," "wan," perhaps "yellowish"—the ancestor of "ochre."

20   *The sudden sight of a snake causes pallor.* The verb is *chlōrotēta*, from *chlōros*, "pale or green," of which more later.

20   *Odysseus strings his great bow. the skin* (or complexion) changed color, *chrōs / etrapeto.*

20   *Pale fear. Chlōron deos.*

21   *Maimonides*. From *Regimen of Health*. Cited in Abraham Joshua Heschel, *Maimonides: A Biography*, trans. Joachim Neugroschel. (New York: Farrar, Straus & Giroux, 1982), 127.

21   *Dante. Inferno*, book 5, lines 130–131. "Per più fiate li occhi ci sospinse / quella lettura, e scolorocci il viso."

21   *Henry V*. Act IV, Chorus, lines 41–42.

21   *In hemorrhage patients develop a pale color.* From *Epidemics II*, in Wesley D. Smith, ed. and trans. *Hippocrates:* Volume VII (Cambridge, MA: Harvard

University Press, 1994), 34–35. The Greek word is *ekchloiountai*, which could be rendered as "becomes pale or green." More later.

21   *Two brothers who bleed. Epidemics IV*. In Smith, 116–17. The word is *chloōdeis*—pale or green, again.

22   *Death rides a pale horse*. Revelation 6:8.

22   *Wyndham Lewis. Paleface: The Philosophy of the "Melting-Pot"* (New York: Haskell House Publishers, 1929, reprint 1969).

22   *Philip Rahv*. Reprinted in *Image and Idea: Fourteen Essays on Literary Themes* (Norfolk, CT: New Directions, 1949).

22   *Ochwiay Biano*. C. G. Jung, *Memories, Dreams, Reflections*, recorded and edited by Aniela Jaffé, translated by Richard and Clara Winston (New York: Vintage, 1965), 248.

22   *Romeo and Juliet*. The first quote is from Act II, scene ii, lines 85–86. The second is from Act II, scene v, line 70.

23   *The Wife of Bath. The Canterbury Tales*, General Prologue, lines 458–60. In contemporary spelling,

> Bold was her face, and red of hue,
> She was a worthy woman all her life
> Husbands at church door she had five.

The red-faced male counterpart is the lecherous Summoner, "That hadde a fyr-redde cherubinnes face" (Prologue, line 624).

23   *Esau*. Genesis 25:25.

23   *Chaucer's Franklin. The Canterbury Tales*, General Prologue, lines 332–33.

> Of his complexion he was sanguine.
> Well loved he in the morning some bread in wine.

23   *The porter. Macbeth*, Act II, scene iii, lines 23–25.

24   *The shipmaster*. From *Billy Budd, Sailor, and Other Stories* (New York: Penguin Classics, 1967), 323.

24   *The form of Billy Budd*. Pages 354–55.

24   *Ovid. The Art of Love*, book III, line 74.

24   *Villon. Le Testament*, l. 962. "Vous, laide, sans colour." In another poem, he bequeaths to the same woman, or perhaps some other, his heart, in a box, "pale, piteous, dead and numb." *Le Lais*, ll. 76–7. "mon cuer enchassié / Palle, piteux, mort et transy." François Villon, *The Poems of François Villon*, translated with an introduction and notes by Galway Kinnell (Boston: Houghton Mifflin Company, 1977).

24   *Cosmetics. The Art of Love*, book III, lines 199–200.

25   *Villon*. "Ballade (Je cognois bien mouches en let.)" The final stanza reads:

> Prince, je congnois tout en somme
> Je congnois coulourez et blesmes
> Je congnois Mort quit tout sonsomme
> Je congnois tout fors que moy mesmes.

25   *Song of Songs* 5:10. The Hebrew words are *tzach* (dazzling white,

sunlit, bright, clear, hot) and *adom* (red, red-cheeked, a red thing, red color), the latter related to the words *adam* (man), *adamah* (earth), and *dam* (blood). *Adom* is the same word used to describe Esau in Genesis 25:25. The definitions are from *Langenscheidt's Dictionary of Biblical Hebrew*; the analysis is by Michael S. Diamond, M.D., personal communication, June 16, 2007.

3: THE MALICE SICKLE

27   *Sickle cell and malaria resistance.* One analysis of the Yoruba of Nigeria concluded that the likelihood of surviving to adulthood was significantly increased (by about 14 percent) if a child carried one sickle gene (AS heterozygote), but markedly reduced (by about 84 percent) if he carried two (SS homozygote). W.F. Bodmer and L.L. Cavalli-Sforza, *Genetics, Evolution, and Man* (San Francisco: W. H. Freeman, 1976).

27   *Senegal.* Fullwiley ,D. "Biosocial Suffering: Order and Illness in Urban West Africa." *BioSocieties* (2006):421–38.

28   *Herrick.* Savitt, T.L., & Goldberg, M.F. "Herrick's 1910 Case Report of Sickle Cell Anemia: The Rest of the Story, *Journal of the American Medical Association* 261 (1989):266–71.

28   *Changed molecule.* The discovery, and the term "molecular disease," was coined by Linus Pauling, later a Nobel laureate in Chemistry and then in Peace.

29   *Criminal prosecution.* Reidenberg, M.M., & Willis, O. "Prosecution of Physicians for Prescribing Opioids to Patients." *Clinical Pharmacology and Therapeutics* 81, no. 6 (2007): 797–8 (accessed April 15, 2007, ahead of print). *See also* John Tierney, "Trafficker or Healer? And Who's the Victim?" *New York Times*, March 27, 2007.

29   *80,000 Americans.* Press release, Sickle Cell Disease Association of America, September 27, 2006. htttp://www.prnewswire.com/cgi-bin /stories.pl?ACCT=104&STORY=/www/story/09-27-2006 /0004440522 &EDATE=.

30   *Saturn.* So Susan Sontag writes of Walter Benjamin, in her essay "Under the Sign of Saturn," collected in the book of the same title. Her antecedents are Rudolph and Margot Wittkower, *Born Under Saturn: The Character and Conduct of Artists* (1963); and Raymond Klibansky, Erwin Panofsky and Fritz Saxl, *Saturn and Melancholy: Studies in the History of Natural Philosophy, Religion, and Art* (1964). The latter exceptional book was to be published in Germany in 1939, after its authors had fled to Britain, but the war first delayed publication and then destroyed the plates entirely. Only the book's translation into English, and some additional modifications, allowed for its long overdue publication in 1964.

32   *Senegal.* Fullwiley, D. "Discriminate Biopower and Everyday Biopolitics: Views on Sickle Cell Testing in Dakar," *Medical Anthropology* 23 (2004):157–94.

32   *Spreading.* Wailoo, K. "Genetic Marker of Segregation: Sickle Cell Anemia, Thalassemia, and Racial Ideology in American Medical Writing 1920–1950." *History and Philosophy of the Life Sciences* 18 (1996):305–20.

33   *The slaying of Orpheus.* Drawing after a classical Attic red figure vase attributed to the Niobid Painter. Museum of Fine Arts, Boston (Boston 90.156).

4: THE GREEN SICKNESSE

37   *Sappho.* Fragment 31.

37   *Lady Macbeth. Macbeth,* Act I, scene vii, lines 35–37.

38   *Lange.* "*De Morbo Virgeneo,*" in *Medicinalium epistolarum miscellanea* (Basle: Welchelus, 1554), reprinted in Ralph H. Major, ed. and trans., *Classic Descriptions of Disease. 3rd Edition* (Springfield, IL: Charles C. Thomas, 1932).

38   *English authors.* Helen King, *Disease of Virgins* (New York: Routledge, 2004).

38   *Robert Greene* was an Elizabethan writer of prose, poetry, and drama, best known today as the author of *Friar Bacon and Friar Bungay* (c. 1589). The citation is from his prose fiction *Mamillia: A Mirrour or Looking-Glasse for the Ladies of England* (1583). It was Greene who seemed to accuse Shakespeare of plagiarism, calling him "an upstart Crow beautified with our feathers" with a "Tygers hart wrapt in a Players hyde." (*Groatsworth of Wit*, 1592).

39   *Falstaff. The Second Part of King Henry IV,* Act IV, scene iii, lines 87–91. The play was probably written about 1598.

39   *Jean Varandal, De morbis et affectibus mulierum* (Lyons: B Vincent, 1619), 4–5 (cited in King, 148).

39   *Diseases of Young Women.* The Greek title is *Peri Parthenion,* raising the never settled question of how to render the crucial word *parthénos:* young woman, girl, virgin, maiden. Here the main sense seems to be "virgin" in the modern American sense, as it discusses ailments that are cured by marriage and sexual intercourse. The brief treatise has not, to the best of my knowledge, been translated into English but may be read in the French version of Paul-Émile Littré, whose famous translations of Hippocrates, completed in 1862, were for many years the most authoritative in any modern European language. "*Des maladies des jeunes filles,*" in *Hippocrate, Oeuvres Complètes,* Volume 8, 464–71.

    The Parthenon of the Athenian Acropolis is so named, of course, in dedication to Athena Parthenos, the goddess in her capacity as Virgin, a power to be reckoned with.

39   *Sydenham. Processus Integri,* "Chapter XLVI: On the Green-Sickness." *The Works of Thomas Sydenham, M.D., Translated from the Latin Edition of Dr. Greenhill with a Life of the Author, by R.G. Latham, M.D.* (London: The Sydenham Society, 1818), reprinted by the Classics of Medicine Library, 1979.

40   *Putrid humors.* Sydenham, *Epistolary Dissertation*, sections 91–98.

40   *Montesquieu (Charles de Secondat, baron de Montesquieu).* "Letter 143," from *The Persian Letters,* trans. John Davidson (London: Gibbings & Company, 1899); and http://www.wm.edu/history/rbsche/plp/.

40   *Pietro Aretino (1492–1556),* the great Italian humanist and satirist, also wrote the *Sonetti Lussuriosi* ("Lewd Sonnets") and the *Ragionamenti* ("The Dialogues"), in which an old courtesan teaches the trade to a novice. Jacob Burckhardt calls him "the greatest railer of modern times." *The Civilization of the Renaissance in Italy,* Volume 1, trans. Ludwig Geiger and Walther Götz (New York: Harper & Row, 1929), 170. Thomas Sanchez, S.J. (1550–1610) is the author of *Disputationes de sancti matrimonii sacramento* ("Disputations on The Holy Sacrament of Matrimony") *The Catholic Encyclopedia,* http://www.newadvent.org /cathen /index.html.

41   *Doctor Johnson.* The Johnson Dictionary Project. http:www.fab24 .net/jd100203/index_.html.

41   *Bleichsucht.* For example, in the dictionary of the philologist Brothers Grimm, "*Bleichsucht*" is defined as "*f. chlorosis, morbus virgineus.*" *Deutsches Wörterbuch von Jacob Grimm und Wilhelm Grimm* (Leipzig: S. Hirzel, 1854–1960), and http://www.woerterbuchnetz .de/woerterbuecher/dwb.

41   *Baudelaire.* "Le Soleil," from *Fleurs du Mal* (1857). The poet describes the sun as "Ce père nourricier, ennemi des chloroses," l. 9. "This life-giving sun, enemy of chloroses."

42   *Louis-Ferdinand Céline, Guignol's Band,* trans. Bernard Frechtman and Jack T. Nile (New York: New Directions, 1954).

42   *Google.com* and *Amazon.com.* The figures are from April 28, 2007.

42   *Standard dictionary. An Intermediate Greek-English Lexicon, Founded upon the Seventh Edition of Liddell and Scott's Greek-English Lexicon* (1889; reprint, Oxford: Oxford University Press, 1997).

42   *Prognostic.* In *Hippocrates, with an English Translation by W.H.S. Jones,* Vol. II (Cambridge, MA: Harvard University Press, 1923).

43   *Color symbolism.* For example, Ivor H. Evans, ed. *Brewer's Dictionary of Phrase and Fable.* Centenary Edition, revised. (New York: Harper & Row, 1981).

43   *Wedding dresses.* Ian Paterson, *A Dictionary of Colour* (London: Thorogood Publishing, 2004), 191.

43   *Demeter Chloe.* Pausanias, *Description of Greece,* Book 1, Chapter 22, Section 3.

46   *Portrait of a young girl.* Drawing after a Pompeian fresco painting of Sappho, now in the National Archaeological Museum, Naples.

5: Anemia's Old Tale

47   *The wounding of Aphrodite.* The *Iliad,* Book V, lines 339–42. This is the first appearance of a word resembling the modern "anemia." The

concept behind the word is very different from ours.

47   *Hippocratic facies. Prognostic*, in *Hippocrates, with an English Translation by W.H.S. Jones*,Vol. II (Cambridge, MA: Harvard University Press, 1923).

47   *Whitishness.* The Greek phrase is *"to hypoleukon." Epidemics III*, in *Hippocrates, with an English Translation by W.H.S. Jones*, Vol. I (Cambridge, MA: Harvard University Press, 1923). 254–5.

48   *White Phlegm. Affections*, in *Hippocrates, Vol. V, with an English Translation by Paul Potter* (Cambridge, MA: Harvard University Press, 1988). Elsewhere (*Diseases II*), the disease White Phlegm seems to reflect some edematous state. The one that comes nearest, in modern terms, is the kidney disease called nephrotic syndrome—or perhaps the parasitic infection schistosomiasis.

48   *Aristotle. History of Animals*, Book III, Part 19, trans. D'Arcy Wentworth Thompson.University of Adelaide Library. http://wwwetext.library.adelaide.edu.au/a/aristotle.

49   *Ayurveda.* G.D. Singhal and T.J.S. Patterson. *Synopsis of Ayurveda: Based on a Translation of the Suśruta Samhitā (The Treatise of Suśruta)* (Delhi: Oxford University Press, 1993). The pertinent sections of the *Suśruta Samhitā* are I.1 and VI.44.The explications of the humors come from the authors' introduction, "A Note on Indian Medicine."

49   *Pallor also occurs. Suśruta Samhitā*, I.14.30.

50   *Ibn Sīnā. The Canon of Medicine: Adapted by Laleh Bakhtiar from Translations of Volume I by O. Cameron Gruner and Mazar H. Shah, Correlated with the Arabic by Jay R. Crook with Notes by O. Cameron Gruner* (Chicago: KAZI Publications, 1999).The citation is from Part III, Section 11.4.4. Ibn Sīnā does go on to say a few words about greenness; these seem to intersect the concept jaundice rather than chlorosis.

50   *I am different. Paracelsus: Selected Writings*, ed. Jolande Jacobi, trans. Norbert Guterman (New York: Pantheon Books, 1951).

51   *Toxicities of mercury in the treatment of syphilis.* These are vividly depicted by Alphonse Daudet in *La Doulou*, a collection of unfinished notes from the 1880s, translated by Julian Barnes as *In the Land of Pain* (New York: Knopf, 2003).

51   *Erythrocytes.* Some say that the first to observe red blood cells was the Pisan physician Marcello Malpighi, who published his *Micrographia* in 1665. He was certainly the first to describe capillaries, thus revealing the final secret in the circulation of the blood.

52   *Haller. Dr. Albrecht Haller's Physiology: being a course of lectures upon the visceral anatomy and vital oeconomy of human bodies. . . : compiled for the use of the University of Gottingen: now illustrated with useful remarks: with an history of medicine: and with a nosology, or doctrine of diseases.* Cited in Camille Dreyfus, *Some Milestones in the History of Hematology* (New York: Grune & Stratton, 1957).

52   *Apparatuses.* For example, Karl von Vierordt (1818–1884).

52   *Red cell count.* Williams Gowers, *On the Numeration of the Red Corpuscles* (1877). Paul Ehrlich and A. Lazarus, *Anaemia.*

53   *Studies conclude.* Steven McGee, *Evidence-Based Physical Diagnosis* (Philadelphia: Saunders, 2001), 96–9.

6: WHAT THE DOCTOR IS THINKING

60   *Galen.* "The Art of Medicine," in *Galen: Selected Works,* P.N. Singer, ed. and trans. (Oxford: Oxford University Press, 1997), 358.

60   *Social dominance and control.* Above all, the work of Michel Foucault.

60   *Political arithmetic. Encyclopaedia Britannica,* 11th ed., s.v. "Statistics." For example, Sir William Petty, *Five Essays in Political Arithmetic* (1683).

62   *Thomson.* "Electrical Units of Measurement" (lecture delivered at the Institution of Civil Engineers, May 3, 1883), in *Popular Lectures and Addresses. Volume 1: Constitution of Matter* (New York: Macmillan & Co., 1891), 80.

62   *Erhlich. Anaemia* (New York: Rebman, 1910).

7: DIAGNOSTIC CEREMONIES

66   *spinach and iron:* see notes to Chapter 1.

66   *Recommended Daily Allowance of iron.* Institute of Medicine, Food and Nutrition Board, "Dietary Reference Intakes for Vitamin A, Vitamin K, Arsenic, Boron, Chromium, Copper, Iodine, Iron, Manganese, Molybdenum, Nickel, Silicon, Vanadium and Zinc" (Washington, DC: National Academy Press, 2001).

67   *A little homework.* United States National Institutes of Health, Office of Dietary Supplements, http://wwwods.od.nih.gov/factsheets/iron.asp.

67   *Pica.* Woywodt, A. and Kiss, A. "Geophagia: The History of Earth-Eating," *Journal of the Royal Society of Medicine* 95 (2002):143–46.

68   *Don Quixote.* Chapter 33, "comer tierra, yeso, carbón y otras cosas peores."

68   *Scrutiny.* Vermeer, D.E. and Frate, D.A., "Geophagia in Rural Mississippi: Environmental and Cultural Contexts and Nutritional Implications," *American Journal of Clinical Nutrition* 32 (1979):2129–35.

68   *Pharmacologic benefits.* Vermeer, D.E. and Ferrell, R.E., Jr., "Nigerian Geophagical Clay: A Traditional Antidiarrheal Pharmaceutical," *Science* 227 (1985):634–36.

77   *Commercial laboratories.* Quest Diagnostics, for example, offers the "Ashkenazi Jewish Panel." This tests the patient for eight hereditary conditions: Bloom syndrome, Canavan disease, cystic fibrosis, familial dysautonomia, Fanconi anemia Group C, Gaucher disease, Niemann-Pick disease, and Tay-Sachs disease. http://www.questdiagnostics.com.

77   *BRCA genetic testing.* Estimates vary widely. The figures cited are estimates of the National Cancer Institute of the National Institutes of

Health. PDQ Cancer Information Summaries, Genetics, http://www
.cancer.gov/cancertopics/pdq/genetics.

8: SPLEEN

85   *Spleen and sorcery.* Isaac Keango Nyamongo. "Lay People's Responses
     to Illness: An Ethnographic Study of Anti-Malarial Behavior Among
     the Abagusii of Southwestern Kenya." PhD dissertation, University of
     Florida, 1988. http://www.etd.fcla.edu/UF/amd0025/master.pdf.
     See also LeVine, R.A., "Witchcraft and Sorcery in a Gusii Commun-
     ity," in *Witchcraft and Sorcery in East Africa.* Eds. J. Middleton and E. H.
     Winter (New York: Frederick A. Praeger, 1963), 221–55.

86   *The four elements.* These were first articulated by Empedocles, a
     Sicilian Greek of the fifth century BCE, by profession a physician,
     who wrote his philosophy in verse. Their analogues in medicine,
     the four humors, first became a systematic tetrad in the treatise *On
     the Nature of Man*, written in the late fifth century BCE and attrib-
     uted to Hippocrates or to his son-in-law Polybus. The related doc-
     trine of the four temperaments or complexions—the sanguine,
     phlegmatic, choleric, and melancholic character types—had been
     percolating for centuries but was first codified clearly by the
     scholastic philosopher William of Conches (ca. 1100–54). See
     Klibansky, Saxl, and Panofsky, 102ff.

87   *Jaques. As You Like It,* Act IV, scene i.

87   *Aristotle. Problems,* III.1.

87   *Robert Burton, The Anatomy of Melancholy.* Ed. and trans. Floyd Dell
     and Paul Jordan-Smith (New York: Tudor Publishing Company,
     1927), 38ff.

87   *Austen, Pride and Prejudice,* Chapter 27. A favorite phrase of the artist
     Barbara Kilpatrick, who pointed me there.

87   *Baudelaire.* From one of the several poems entitled "Spleen" (*"J'ai plus
     de souvenirs que si j'avais mille ans"*), ll. 15-18. *Les Fleur du Mal* (1857).

88   *Pure art.* Baudelaire, "Philosophic Art," in *The Painter of Modern Life
     and Other Essays*, trans. Jonathan Mayne (New York: Da Capo,
     1986), 205.

88   *Donne. Devotions upon Emergent Occasions*, Meditation VI in *The
     Complete Poetry and Selected Prose of John Donne.* Ed. Charles M.
     Coffin (New York: Modern Library, 1994), 422.

89   *Drawing after Albrecht Dürer.* "Self-portrait with the Yellow-Spot,"
     Bremen, Kunsthalle. The figure comes from a drawing that the artist
     sent a distant physician, demonstrating the site of his pain. He indi-
     cates the area of the spleen, highlighted in yellow. G.D. Schott. "The
     Sick Dürer—A Renaissance Prototype Pain Map," *British Medical
     Journal* 329 (2004):1492–93.

9: MARROW

90   *Hercules. Metamorphoses*, 9.174–5.

90   *Pythagoras. Metamorphoses,* 15.389–90.

90   Sir *Thomas Browne, Hydriotaphia: Urn Burial, or A Brief Discourse of the Sepulcral Urns lately found in Norfolk,* in *Religio Medici, Hydriotaphia and The Garden of Cyrus,* ed. R.H.A. Robbins (Oxford: Clarendon Press, 2001), 117.

91   *Rabelais. Gargantua,* in *The Complete Works of François Rabelais,* Donald M. Frame, trans. (Berkeley: University of California Press, 1991), 4.

91   *Proverbs.* King James Version, 3.7–8.

91   *The Joints and Marrow.* Hebrews, 4.12

92   *Boy of Kenya.* Isaac G.L.L., "The Activities of Early African Hominids, in *Human Origins—Louis Leakey and the East African Evidence,* Glynn L. L. Isaac and Elizbeth R. McCown, eds. (Menlo Park, CA:W.A. Benjamin, 1976).

92   *English cookery and medicine.* Thomas Austin, ed. *Two Fifteenth-Century Cookery-Books* (London: Early English Text Society, 1888). Thomas Elyot, *The Castel of Helth,* 1541 (reprint New York: Scholars' Facsimiles & Reprints, 1936).

92   *fat of the land.* Genesis 45.18.

92   *Chelev. chet, lamed, vet.* Michael S. Diamond, M.D., personal communication, January 6, 2007.

92   *Fat things full of marrow.* Isaiah 25.6.

92   *Marrow and Fatness.* Psalms 63.5.

92   *Dido. Aeneid* 4.66. "*Est mollis flamma medullas.*"

92   *Venus and Adonis.* line 142. Astonishing that any could resist her.

92   *Catullus.* Carmen 100. "*Cum vesana meas torreret flamma medullas.*" Compare the Virgil passage above.

93   *Parolles. All's Well that Ends Well,* Act II, scene iii.

93   *Marrow-bones and prayer.* Yeats, "Adam's Curse," in *The Collected Poems of W.B. Yeats.* (New York: Macmillan, 1933), 78. The word sometimes transmogrifies into "mary-bones," as in Thomas Nashe, *The Unfortunate Traveller* (1594).

93   *Yeats.* "Prayer for Old Age." (New York: Macmillan, 1933), 78

93   *Rilke.* Untitled fragment from *Collected Works,* Vol. 2.

10: DISEASES OF THE BLOOD

94   *Shakespeare's sovereign thrones. Twelfth Night, or What You Will,* Act I, scene i. John Donne, born a few years later but made quite differently, assigns sovereignty to the heart—even well past his tempestuous youth. *Devotions upon Emergent Occasions,* Meditation XI.

94   *Tripartite soul.* Plato, *The Republic,* and especially *Timaeus.*

95   *Eisenhower.* Clarence G. Lasby, *Eisenhower's Heart Attack: How Ike Beat*

Heart Disease and Held on to the Presidency (Lawrence: University of Kansas Press, 1997).

96   *Liver-spleen symmetry.* Aristotle, *On the Parts of Animals*, III.7. At the same time, he considered the two lungs to be a single organ, joined in the middle.

97   *Maimonides. The Regimen of Health*, in "Moses Maimonides' Two Treatises on the Regimen of Health," *Transactions of the American Philosophical Society*, New Series, Volume 54, Part 4. Translated and edited by Ariel Bar-Sela, M.D., Hebbel E. Hoff, M.D., and Elias Faris. (Philadelphia: The American Philosophical Society, 1964), 20.

97   *The liver in France.* Lynn Payer, *Medicine and Culture* (New York: Penguin, 1989).

97   *Aristotle. On the Parts of Animals*, II.7.

98   *Second childishness. As You Like It*, Act II, scene vii, lines 166–67.

98   *Shrine to Mens.* Livy, *The History of Rome from its Foundation*, 22.9–10.

100   *Pneuma* is the Greek term for breath, also spirit, also wind. In the *Septuagint*, the Greek translation of the Jewish Bible that became the basic source of the Christian Old Testament, the spirit of God that moves across the water is "*pneuma*" (Genesis 1.2). "*Arwah*" is the Arabic equivalent, "*spiritus*" the Latin, if such terms can ever have true intercultural equivalents.

100   *Aceldama.* Matthew 27:5–8, Acts I, 16–19.

101   *Cain.* Genesis 4:11.

101   *Blood of Abel.* Matthew 23:35.

101   *Erinyes.* Hesiod, *Theogony*.

101   *Aeschylus, The Libation Bearers*, Act II, 67–70.

102   *Tuberculosis.* For this view, Thomas Mann, *The Magic Mountain*.

102   *Chronic lymphocytic leukemia and its name.* Hoffbrand, A. Victor, and Hamblin, T.J., "Is 'leukemia' an Appropriate Label for All Patients Who Meet the Diagnostic Criteria of Chronic Lymphocytic Leukemia?" *Leukemia Research* 31 (2007):273–75.

11: ANEMIA WORLD

104   *World Health Organization.* "Joint Statement by the World Health Organization and the United Nations Children's Fund, Focusing on Anaemia: Towards an Integrated Approach for Effective Anaemia Control," http://www.who.int/topics/anaemia/en/who_unicef-anaemiastatement.pdf.

104   *World's population.* United States Census Bureau. World Population Information. http://www.census.gov/ipc/www/world.html.

104   *Côte d'Ivoire.* Asobayire, F.S., Adou, P., Davidsson, L., Cook, J.D., and Hurrell, R.F., "Prevalence of Iron Deficiency with and without Concurrent Anemia in Population Groups with High Prevalences

of Malaria and Other Infections: A study in Côte d'Ivoire," *American Journal of Clinical Nutrition* 74 (2001):776–82.

105 *Anemia in hunters and farmers.* Hart, G.D., "Ancient diseases of the blood," in *Blood Pure and Eloquent*, Maxwell M. Wintrobe, ed. (New York: McGraw-Hill, 1980).

105 *Early days of civilization.* Roy Porter, *The Greatest Benefit to Mankind: A Medical History of Humanity* (New York: W.W. Norton, 1997), 18–19.

106 *Intestinal worms.* World Health Organization, "Schistosomiasis and Soil-Transmitted Helminth Infections—Preliminary Estimates of the Number of Children Treated with Albendazole or Mebendazole," *Weekly Epidemiological Record* 81 (2006):145–64. http://www.who .int/wer.

106 *Proximity.* Porter, *The Greatest Benefit to Mankind.*

107 *Tertian and quartan fevers.* Hippocrates, *Epidemics III*; *Nature of Man*, xv.

107 *Dante. Inferno* 17.85–7.

107 *Verga.* The author (1840–1922) is best known for his *verismo* portrayal of rural Sicilian life and above all for his 1880 story "Cavalleria Rusticana," on which the Mascagni opera was based.

107 *Slime and marshes. Humors* 12.

107 *Varro. "Advertendum etiam, siqua erunt loca palustria . . . et quod crescunt animalia quaedam minuta, quae non possunt oculi consequi, et per aera intus in corpus per os ac nares perveniunt atque efficiunt difficilis morbos." De re rustica* [On Rustic Matters], Chapter 12, http://www.intratext.com /X/LAT0056.HTM.

108 *A million children.* World Heath Organization, Global Malaria Programme. http://www.malaria.who.int.

108 *Half the world's population.* Worth Health Organization, World Malaria Report 2005. http://www.rbm.who.int/wmr2005.

109 *1.3%.* Sachs J.D. "Macroeconomics and Health: Investing in Health for Economic Development." *Report of the Commission on Macroeconomics and Health* (Geneva: World Health Organization, December 2001).

109 *Neolithic.* James H. Mielke, Lyle W. Konigsberg, John H. Relethford, *Human Biological Variation* (New York: Oxford University Press, 2006), 150.

109 *Frontier malaria in the Amazon.* Caldas de Castro, M., Monte-Mór, R.L., Sawyer, D.O., and Singer, B.H., "Malaria Risk on the Amazon Frontier." *Proceedings of the National Academy of Science* 103 (2006):2452–57.

110 *Malaria in the U.S.* Eliades, M.J., Shah, S., Nguyen-Dinh, P., Newman, R.D., Barber, A.M., Nguyen-Dinh, P., Roberts, J.M., Mali, S., Parise, M.E., Barber, A.M. and Steketee, R. "Malaria Surveillance—United States, 2003." *Morbidity and Mortality Weekly Report* 54 (2005):25–40.

111 *The tripartite division* of medical therapies into medication, surgery

and talk is very old, dating at least to the Avestan texts of ancient Persia. Émile Benveniste. La doctrine médicale des Indo-Européens. *Revue de l'Histoire des Religions* 130 (1945) 5–12.

12: IRON

113   *The great life formula.* Oxygen and glucose combine to yield vital energy and two waste products, the gas carbon dioxide and water. This process, called aerobic metabolism, provides the body's energy. The opposite process is photosynthesis, in which plant cells combine carbon dioxide and water, using the sun's energy, to create glucose and a waste product, oxygen. This is the ultimate source of all life energy, deriving ultimately from the sun. The formula is a circle.

The triangular marriage of oxygen, iron, and life goes back very far. Virtually all gaseous oxygen on earth is the excretory product of plant life. In the primeval seas, oxygen excreted by algae combined with dissolved iron to form oxides, a process called oxidation. These iron oxides settled to the ocean floor and formed the geologic deposits that we call iron ore.

114   *People do not eat stones.* Unless they do—the curious behavior called pica or geophagia is discussed in Chapter 7.

114   *Eating or drinking blood.* Alan Davidson, *The Oxford Companion to Food* (New York: Oxford University Press, 1999), 81–2. Early American cooking, less fastidious in the days before microwave dinners and takeout pizza, offered such recipes as the following for blood pudding: "Take your Indian meal (according to the quantity you wish to make), and scald it with boiled milk or water, then stir in your blood, straining it first, mince the hog's lard and put it in the pudding, then season it with treacle and pounded penny-royal to your taste, put it in a bag and let it boil six or seven hours." Susannah Carter, *The Frugal Housewife, or Complete Woman Cook* (New York: G. & R. Waite, 1803). This text and many others are reprinted, with introductory commentaries, at Feeding America: The Historic American Cookbook Project, sponsored by Michigan State University, http://www.digital.lib.msu.edu/projects/cookbooks. I am grateful to Anne Mendelson for pointing me there.

114   *Jugo de carne.* Zarela Martínez, personal communication, July 10, 2007.

114   *Themistocles.* Plutarch, *Lives of the Noble Greeks and Romans*, "Themistocles"; Valerius Maximus, *Nine Books of Memorable Deeds and Sayings*, 5.6.

115   *Voltaire. Philosophical Dictionary*, entry on "Poisonings."

115   *Healing cults.* Encyclopaedia Britannica 2008 Ultimate Reference Suite, s.v. "healing cults."

115   *Austen's Bath.* For example, as portrayed in *Northanger Abbey* and *Sanditon.*

115 *Ibn Sīnā. Canon of Medicine*, 10.8.2. and 10.11.1. In Bakhtiar's translation, 229 and 237.

116 *Suśruta Samhitā.* I.38, in *Synopsis of Ayurveda*, 35–6.

116 *Treatment with iron. Suśruta Samhitā,* VI.44, in *Synopsis of Ayurveda*, 79–80.

116 *Chomwe.* Young, S.L. and Ali, S.M. "Linking Traditional Treatments of Maternal Anaemia to Iron Supplement Use: An Ethnographic Case Study from Pemba Island, Zanzibar," *Maternal & Child Nutrition* 1 (2006):51–58.

116 *Dioscorides.* Robert T. Gunther, ed., *The Greek Herbal of Dioscorides, Illustrated by a Byzantine A.D. 512, Englished by John Goodyer A.D. 1655, Edited and First Printed A.D. 1933* (London and New York: Hafner Publishing Company, 1968).

117 *Magic.* We are not speaking, of course, of conjuring, witchcraft, sorcery, necromancy, sleight of hand, levitations, hocus-pocus, or abracadabra.

117 *Telchines.* Strabo, *Geography*, 14.2.7. Diodorus Siculus, *Library*, 5.3. Callimachus, *Hymn to Delos*, line 31.

117 *Dactyls.* Diodorus Siculus, *Library*, 5.4. Jung further reports that the Dactyls were the first Wise Men and the teachers of Orpheus. C.G. Jung, *Symbols of Transformation: An Analysis of the Prelude to a Case of Schizophrenia.* Trans. R.F.C. Hull (Princeton: Princeton University Press, 1976), 176–7.

117 *World's oldest mine.* George J. Coakley, *The Mineral Industry of Swaziland.* United States Geological Survey, http://www.minerals .usgs.gov. Dart, R.A. and Beaumont, P., "Evidence of Iron Ore Mining in Southern Africa in the Middle Stone Age." *Current Anthropology* 10 (1969):127–28.

118 *Bomvu. Zulu-English/English-Zulu Online Dictionary.* http://www .isizulu.net.

118 *Prehistoric ocher.* Henshilwood, C.S., d'Errico, F., Yates, R., Jacobs, Z., Tribolo, C., et al., "Emergence of Modern Human Behavior: Middle Stone Age Engravings from South Africa," *Science* 295 (2002):1278–80.

118 *Incised ocher.* Drawing after a photograph of the object by Professor Henshilwood, presented in a lecture by Ian Tattersall at The Metropolitan Museum of Art, New York, on the occasion of the symposium "Genesis: Exploration of Origins" on March 7, 2003, http://www.metmuseum.org/special/Genesis/tattersall_lecture .asp.

118 *European cave paintings.* Jean-Marie Chauvet, Eliette Brunel Deschamps, Christian Hillaire, *Dawn of Art: The Chauvet Cave (The Oldest Known Paintings in the World)* (New York: Abrams, 1996).

118 *Kapthurin Formation.* McBrearty, S. and Brooks, A.S., "The Revolution That Wasn't: A New Interpretation of the Origin of Modern Human

behavior," *Journal of Human Evolution* 39 (2000):453–563.

119   *Egyptian and Roman painting.* François Delamare and Bernard Guineau, *Colors: The Story of Dyes and Pigments.* Trans. Sophie Hawkes. (New York: Harry N. Abrams, Inc., 2000), 20–33.

119   *Red Ocher Culture.* Franklin Folsom and Mary Elting Folsom, *America's Ancient Treasures: A Guide to Archeological Sites and Museums in the United States and Canada,* 3rd Rev. Ed. (Albuquerque: University of New Mexico Press, 1983), 250–51.

119   *The Egyptians.* Encyclopaedia Britannica, 11th Edition, Vol. 9, 68–69.

119   *Ba-n-pet.* H.R. Hall, *Note on the Early Use of Iron in Egypt* (London: Anthropological Institute, 1903).

119   *Indo-European.* Calvert Watkins, ed. *The American Heritage Dictionary of Indo-European Roots.* 2nd Ed. (Boston, New York: Houghton Mifflin, 2000), 23. See also the editor's introduction, "Indo-European and the Indo-Europeans, p. xxxi. The root, which originally seems to relate to passion in various forms, also gives rise to Latin *ira* ("anger," cognates "irate," etc.); to Greek *hieros* ("filled with the divine," cognates "hieroglyphics," etc.); and to Greek *oistros* ("gadfly, something causing madness," cognates "estrus, estrogen").

120   *Golden Age and thereafter.* Hesiod, *Works and Days,* ll. 106ff. The myth of an idyllic epoch preceding one's own is very ancient, recorded in the world's oldest extant literature, that of the Sumerians, who ruled Mesopotamia in the fourth and third millennia BCE. Samuel Noah Kramer, *Sumerian Mythology* (New York: Harper & Brothers, 1961). Recorded in cuneiform on clay tablets, any further unexcavated records of our oldest known literature have probably been destroyed in the recent U.S.-Iraqi war.

120   *Race of iron.* Hesiod, *Works and Days,* ll. 176–8.

120   *Men first used iron.* M.I. Finley, *Early Greece: The Bronze and Archaic Ages* (New York: W.W. Norton & Company, 1980).

120   *Ovid. Metamorphoses.* Trans. Rolfe Humphries (Bloomington: Indiana University Press, 1955), 5–15.

120   *Donne.* "The First Anniversarie: An Anatomie of the World," line 426.

120   *Persian mythology.* Mircea Eliade, *The Myth of the Eternal Return.* Trans. Willard R. Trask (Princeton: Princeton University Press, 1959), 124–6.

121   *James George Frazer. The Golden Bough.* A new abridgement from the second and third editions, edited by Robert Fraser (New York: Oxford University Press, 1994), 180–3.

121   *Thales.* So says Aristotle, *De Anima* 405a, in *The Basic Works of Aristotle,* Richard McKeon, ed. (New York: Random House, 1941), 541.

121   *All things have souls.* G.S. Kirk, J.E. Raven and M. Schofield, *The Presocratic Philosophers,* 2nd Edition (Cambridge: Cambridge University Press, 1983), 95.

122 Marsilio Ficino. *The Book of Life*. Trans. Charles Boer (Woodstock, CT: Spring Publications, 1980), 133.

122 Pliny the Elder. *Natural History, a Selection*. Trans. John F. Healy (New York: Penguin Books, 2004), 224.

122 Galen. *On the Natural Faculties* 1.14.

123 Renaissance herbal pharmacy. Giambattista della Porta, *Magica Naturalis*, Book 1, Chapter 7. The anonymous English translation of 1658 may be found at http://www.homepages.tscnet.com/omard 1/jportat2.html.

123 Europe's first scientific society. The *Academia Secretorum Naturae* (Academy of the Secrets of Nature), nicknamed the *Otiosi* (Men of Leisure), flourished from 1560 until closed by the Inquisition in 1578. Its successor, the *Accademia dei Lincei* (Academy of Lynxes, founded 1603), included Galileo among its members. These were the forefathers of the *Académie Française* (1635) and the Royal Society (1660).

123 Whirlwind and volcano. "Paracelsus the Physician," in C.G. Jung, *The Spirit in Man, Art, and Literature*. Trans. R.F.C. Hull (Princeton: Bollingen, 1966), 13.

124 Vulcan. *Paracelsus: Selected Writings*, 167.

124 Disease derives from corruption. See, for example, Franciscus Mercurius van Helmont, *One hundred fifty three chymical aphorisms. Briefly containing whatsoever belongs to the chymical science. Done by the labour and study of Eremita Suburbanus. Printed in Latin at Amsterdam, Octob. 1687. To which are added, some other phylosophick canons or rules pertaining to the Hermetick science. Made English and published for the sake of the sedulous labourers in true chymistry . . . by Chr. Packe. London: for the author, sold by W. Cooper. 1688.* http://www.levity.com/alchemy /153aphor.html. The author's father was Jan Baptista van Helmont, "the father of biochemistry."

125 Geritol and iron-poor, tired blood. The current advertising seems to make no mention of this once-ubiquitous slogan.

125 If a star. P.W. Atkins, *The Period Kingdom: A Journey into the Land of the Chemical Elements* (New York: Basic Books, 1995), Chapter 6.

13: BLOODLETTING

126 Bloodletting. Drawing after a red-figure Attic aryballos, ca. 480–470 BCE, the "Peytel aryballos" (Louvre, CA 2183). This vase predates the birth of Hippocrates by some ten years. The patient looks nervous.

127 Horse sacrifice. Thus testifies the *Rig Veda,* for example I.162.

127 Cock sacrifice. Socrates' last words ask his friend to sacrifice a cock to Asklepios. He posits his death as a victory of health. *Phaedo*, 118.a.

128 Holocaust. "These *un*-eaten sacrifices are characteristic of angry ghosts demanding placation and of a whole class of underworld divinities in

general, divinities who belong to a stratum of thought more primitive than Homer." Jane Ellen Harrison, *Prolegomena to the Study of Greek Religion* (Princeton: Princeton University Press, 1991), 16

129   *Plato. Republic* 8.565d; *Laws* 6.782c. The latter citation is from the translation of A.E. Taylor, in Edith Hamilton and Huntington Cairns, eds., *The Collected Dialogues of Plato* (Princeton: Princeton University Press, 1973).

129   *Pharmakos.* Walter Burkert, *Structure and History in Greek Mythology and Ritual* (Berkeley: University of California Press, 1979).

129   *To bless.* Watkins, p. 9. The Indo-European root is *bhel-*, whose modern derivatives include the English words "blood" and "bless."

129   *Sacrifice as gift.* H. Hubert and Marcel Mauss. *Sacrifice: Its Nature and Function.* Trans. W.D. Halls (London: Routledge, 1964). See also Marcel Mauss, *The Gift: The Form and Reason for Exchange in Archaic Societies.* Trans. W.D. Halls (New York: Norton, 1990).

130   *Shaman.* Mircea Eliade, *Shamanism: Archaic Techniques of Ecstasy.* Trans. Willard R. Trask (Princeton: Princeton University Press, 1972), 216.

130   *Heraclitus.* Fragment 14, in G.S. Kirk, J.E. Raven and M. Schofield, *The Presocratic Philosophers*, 2nd ed. (Cambridge: Cambridge University Press, 1983), 209.

131   *Medieval bloodletting.* Drawing after an image of a woman physician, from an early fifteenth-century English manuscript now found in the British Library.

131   *Maimonides. Moses Maimonides on the Causes of Symptoms.* Ed. J. O. Leibowitz and S. Marcus (Berkeley: University of California Press, 1974), 89. Maimonides' extended views on bloodletting comprise the twelfth treatise of his *Aphorisms*, a selection of medical wisdom gleaned from Greek, Roman, Persian, and Arabic authors. *The Medical Aphorisms of Moses Maimonides*, trans. and ed. by Fred Rosner, M.D. and Suessman Munter, M.D. (New York: Yeshiva University Press, 1970).

131   *Surgeon-barber. Encyclopædia Britannica 2007*, Ultimate Reference Suite, s.v. "barber."

132   *42 million leeches.* Ernst Ackerknecht, *Medicine at the Paris Hospital, 1794-1848* (Baltimore: The Johns Hopkins Press, 1967).

132   *Pedro Calderón de la Barca. El Médico de su Honra.* Biblioteca Virtual Miguel de Cervantes. http://www.cervantesvirtual.com.

132   *Louis, P.C.A.* "Recherche sur les effets de la saignée dans plusieurs maladies inflammatoires," *Archives générales de médecine* 18 (1828): 321–336. The article was expanded into a book and published in 1835. A nice discussion of the issues is found in Morabia, A., "Pierre-Charles-Alexandre Louis and the Evaluation of Bloodletting," The James Lind Library, hhttp://www.jameslindlibrary.org.

133   *Bloodlessness.* The text *Epidemics* describes the following case: "He

drank various drugs to purge upward and downward, and was not benefited. But when he was bled in each arm in turn until he was bloodless, then he was benefited, and freed from the trouble." The phrase rendered as "bloodless" is *exaimos egeneto*, "became bled out." *Epidemics V*, in Wesley D. Smith, ed. and trans. *Hippocrates*, Volume VII (Cambridge, MA: Harvard University Press, 1994), 156–7.

134   *Highly tensed heart.* Nietzsche, *Human, All Too Human: A Book for Free Spirits*, I.138, Trans. R.J. Hollingdale (Cambridge: Cambridge University Press, 1996), 75.

134   *Gift to the gods.* Plato has Socrates say, "Is not sacrifice a giving to the gods, and prayer an asking them to give?" Translation of Lane Cooper. *Euthyphro,* 14c. In Hamilton.

134   *Friendship.* Plato, *Laws*, 6.771.d.

134   *Atonement. The Iliad*, Book 9, line 497.

134   *Burkert. Homo Necans: The Anthropology of Ancient Greek Sacrificial Ritual and Myth.* Trans. Peter Bing (Berkeley: University of California Press, 1983), 135.

134   *The pleasurable shock of survival.* Burkert, 50.

134   *Sacrifice.* For me, the ultimate image is the *Agnus Dei* of Francisco de Zurbarán, a painting of a bound lamb bearing an archaic smile, Museo del Prado.

14: TRANSFUSION

136   *Stefano Infessura. Diario della città di Roma* (Rome: Forzani, 1890).

137   *Lower.* Felts, J.H. "Richard Lower: Anatomist and Physiologist," *Annals of Internal Medicine* 132 (2000):420-3.

137   *Pepys's diary.* Reprinted in its entirety at http://www.pepys.info.

137   *Coga.* The Pepys entry, with commentary, is found at http://www.pepys.info.

138   *Transfusion in intensive care.* Hebert, P.C., Wells, G., Blajchman, M.A., et al., "A Multicenter, Randomized, Controlled Clinical Trial of Transfusion Requirements in Critical Care," *New England Journal of Medicine* 340 (1999):409–17.

138   *Transfusion and race.* See Kenny, M.G., "A Question of Blood, Race, and Politics," *Journal of the History of Medicine and Allied Sciences* 61 (2006):456–491.

138   *"Free and Equal Blues."* Elijah Wald, "Josh White and the Protest Blues," http://www.elijahwald.com/joshprotest.html. The article reproduces the song's lyrics in full.

139   *Tiresias. The Odyssey*, Book 11, line 90.

139   *Bathoy.* http://www.bbc.co.uk/dna/h2g2/A593084. I first heard of the Countess in a footnote to the Cecil Parrott translation of Jaroslav Hašek's novel *The Good Soldier Švejk* (New York: Penguin, 1973), 363 fn.

139   Cosmas and Damian. Their story is recounted in Book V of the *Golden Legend* of Jacobus de Voragine. The complete Caxton translation is found at http://www.fordham.edu/halsall/basis/goldenlegend.

139   Fra Angelico. The Healing of Justinian by Saint Cosmas and Saint Damian, Museo di San Marco, Florence. The image is reproduced at the Web Gallery of Art, http://www.wga.hu.

139   Other Renaissance painters. See, for example, the oil painting on wood attributed to the Master of Los Balbases, Burgos, Spain, ca. 1495. Wellcome Library no. 46009i, reproduced at http://library.wellcome.ac.uk.

15: Is Anemia Good for You?

142   The New York Times. Thursday, November 16, 2006, C1.

142   The New England Journal of Medicine. Drueke, T.B., Locatelli, F., Clyne, N., Eckardt, K.U., Macdougall, I.C., et al., "Normalization of Hemoglobin Level in "Patients with Chronic Kidney Disease and Anemia," *New England Journal of Medicine* 355 (2006):2071–84. Singh, A.K., Szczech, L., Tang, K.L., Barnhart, H., Sapp, S., et al., "Correction of Anemia with Epoetin Alfa in Chronic Kidney Disease," *New England Journal of Medicine* 355 (2006):2085–98.

142   Added twist. Thamer, M., Zhang, Y., Kaufman, J., Cotter, D., Dong, F. and Hernán, M.A., "Dialysis Facility Ownership and Epoetin Dosing in Patients Receiving Hemodialysis," *Journal of the American Medical Association* 297 (2007):1667–74. The point is made forcefully in the accompanying editorial: Coyne, D.W., "Use of Erythropoietin in Chronic Renal Failure," *Journal of the American Medical Association* 297 (2007):1713–6.

144   Some studies. Salonen, J.T., Tuomainen, T.-P., Salonen, R., Lakka, T.A. and Nyyssönen, K., "Donation of Blood Is Associated with Reduced Risk of Myocardial Infarction: The Kuopio Ischaemic Heart Disease Risk Factor Study." *American Journal of Epidemiology* 148 (1998): 445–51. Meyers, D.G., Jensen, K.C. and Menitove, J.E., "A Historical Cohort Study of the Effect of Lowering Body Iron through Blood Donation on Incident Cardiac Events. *Transfusion* 42 (2002) 1135–9.

144   Iron and free radicals. Sullivan, J.L., "Iron and the Sex Difference in Heart Disease Risk," *Lancet* 8233 (1981):1293–94.

16: The Blood of the Medusa

145   Male heroes. Leaving aside, for the present discussion, Freud's argument in his 1922 essay "Medusa's Head" that the Gorgon is a representation of the female genitalia and castration fear; and also Hélène Cixous's call for a new feminist writing in her 1975 essay "The Laugh of the Medusa." So powerful an image conjures many ways. The beauty of myth lies not in the rapid transport from sig-

ndex

nifier to signified, a decodification, but in the resonances and sympathies among the stories themselves.

146   *Poseidon*. Ovid, *Metamorphoses*, Book IV.

146   *Perseus slaying Medusa*. Drawing after a metope from one of the three temples at Selinunte, in Sicily, now found in the National Museum of Palermo. Athena stands by, present but impassive.

146   *Heroic decapitation*. In the Western visual arts, the three preeminent images are the slaying of Medusa, of Holofernes, and of John the Baptist. In opera, these are the subjects of Berlioz's *Benvenuto Cellini* (rather indirectly), Vivaldi's *Juditha Triumphans*, and Strauss's *Salomé*.

147   *Constellations. The Audubon Society Field Guide to the Night Sky* (New York: Knopf, 1991).

147   *Pegasus*. Heroes often ride magic steeds. For Jung, "the hero and his horse seem to symbolize the idea of man and the subordinate sphere of animal instinct. Parallel representations would be Agni on the ram, Wotan on Sleipnir, Ahura-Mazda on Angramainyu, Christ on the ass, Mithras on the bull." C.G. Jung, *Symbols of Transformation*. Trans. R.F.C. Hull (Princeton: Princeton University Press, 1976), 275–6. For Vladimir Propp, the flying hero is an instance of a fundamental component, or "function," of the Russian fairy tale: spatial transference into a different realm, often tinged with magic. *Morphology of the Folktale*, trans. Louis A Wagner (Austin: University of Texas Press, 1968), 50–1.

147   *Athena's shield. The Iliad*, Book 5, line 742.

147   *Agamemnon's shield. The Iliad*, Book 11, line 36.

147   *Vase paintings*. George Henry Chase, *The Shield Devices of the Greeks* (Cambridge, MA: Harvard University Press), 1908.

147   *Hector's Gorgon eyes: The Iliad* Book 8, lines 348–9.

147   *Mask*. Jane Ellen Harrison, *Prolegomena to the Study of Greek Religion* (Cambridge: Cambridge University Press, 1903) 187ff..

147   *Temple of Artemis at Corfu*. Nigel Spivey, *Understanding Greek Sculpture: Ancient Meanings, Modern Readings* (London: Thames & Hudson, 1966), 97–8.

147   *Gilded head of Medusa*. Pausanias, *Description of Greece*, 1.21.3.

147   *Euripides. Ion*, ll. 209–12.

148   *Medusa antefix*. Drawing of an antefix now found in the Princeton University Art Museum, probably manufactured in Taras (the modern Taranto), in the fifth century BCE.

148   *Erichthonius*. Euripides, *Ion*, ll. 999ff.

148   *Goethe. Faust*, Part I, "*Walpurgisnacht*," ll. 4183ff.

148   *medusa / medicine*. Watkins, 52.

149   *Taboo*. In the Navajo tradition, when a man dies, his family seals his hogan, his single-roomed adobe house, with him inside and all his

possessions—then leaves, never to return.

150   *Vedic magic.* Heinrich Zimmer, *Hindu Medicine*, 19.

150   *Medea.* Apollonius of Rhodes, *Argonautica*, III.

150   *Circe. The Odyssey*, Book 10.

150   *Euripides. Andromache*, l. 157.

151   *Ibn Sīnā. Canon of Medicine*, 10.7, 221–2.

151   *Hippocratic Oath.* Rather, the modern physician swears a much-modified, denatured, and bowdlerized version.

152   *Immortal.* The Greek word is *athanatos, a + thanotos*, deathless.

152   *Nietzsche. Human, All Too Human: A Book for Free Spirits.* Trans. R.J. Hollingdale (Cambridge: Cambridge University Press, 1996), 15.

152   *Lucian. The Hall*, "But the beauty of the Gorgons, irresistible in might, won its way to the inmost soul, and wrought amazement and dumbness in the beholder; admiration (so the legend goes) turned him to stone," Trans. H.W. Fowler and F.G. Fowler. htpp://www.sacred-texts.com/cla/luc/wl4/wl400.html.

152   *Pausanias. Description of Greece.*

152   *Christine de Pizan. The City of Ladies.*

152   *Shelley.* "On the Medusa of Leonardo da Vinci in the Florentine Gallery." The poem speaks of the terrible dual nature of horror and beauty, referring to the visage of Medusa, and to certain paintings, and to Leonardo (to whom the painting was wrongfully ascribed). It could have meant medicine in the same breath.

17: THE BIRTH OF CLINICAL TRAGEDY

153   Aeschylus. *Suppliant Women*, ll. 20–3.

156   Hippocrates. *Epidemics.*

156   *The Iliad.* Book I, 1ine 8.

156   *The Oresteia. Agamemnon*, line 192.

156   *The Suppliant Women*, lines 260–70.

156   *Oedipus Tyrannus*, line 25ff.

157   Ovid, *Metamorphoses.* Book 15, lines 622–744.

157   *Pentheus.* Euripides, *The Bacchae.*

157   *Seer.* The myth of Melampus tells how he rescued infant snakes, who licked his ears in gratitude and bestowed him with the powers of seer and physician. Apollodorus, *Library*, 1.9.11.

167   *Laocoön. Aeneid* 2, ll. 199ff.

157   *Spilt blood of Medusa.* As Perseus flew over the Libyan desert with the severed head of Medusa, drops of blood fell on the sand and became or engendered venomous serpents. Lucan calls the story a deceitful fable but recounts it in detail; *Pharsalia* 9.619ff.

158   Whitman. "Reconciliation."